Hospital Joint Ventures Legal Handbook

Max M. Reynolds

JONES AND BARTLETT PUBLISHERS
Sudbury, Massachusetts
BOSTON   TORONTO   LONDON   SINGAPORE

World Headquarters

Jones and Bartlett
  Publishers
40 Tall Pine Drive
Sudbury, MA 01776
978-443-5000
info@jbpub.com
www.jbpub.com

Jones and Bartlett
  Publishers Canada
2406 Nikanna Road
Mississauga,
ON L5C 2W6
CANADA

Jones and Bartlett
  Publishers
  International
Barb House, Barb Mews
London W6 7PA
UK

Library of Congress Cataloging-in-Publication Data

Reynolds, Max.
  Hospital joint ventures legal handbook / Max Reynolds.-- 1st ed.
      p. cm.
  Includes bibliographical references and index.
    ISBN 0-7637-4779-3 (hardcover)
    1. Hospital-physician joint ventures–Law and legislation–United States.
    I. Title.
    KF3825.R49 2004
    344.7303'211–dc22

2003021672

Production Credits
Publisher: Michael Brown
Production Manager: Amy Rose
Associate Editor: Chambers Moore
Production Assistant: Tracey Chapman
Marketing Manager: Joy Stark-Vancs
Marketing Associate: Elizabeth Waterfall
Manufacturing Buyer: Therese Bräuer
Cover Design: Bret Kerr
Composition: Dartmouth Publishing, Inc.
Printing and Binding: Malloy, Inc.
Cover Printing: Malloy, Inc.

Printed in the United States of America
08 07 06 05 04   10 9 8 7 6 5 4 3 2 1

A11417 361923

Dedication

To my wife Toinette. Without her constant encouragement and support, this work would not have been possible.

Table of Contents

Acknowledgments

I owe a debt of gratitude to several individuals for assistance with this work. Chief among them are Guy Collier and Christopher Janney. Guy and Chris are, simply stated, tremendous attorneys and even better mentors. I feel privileged to work with both of them. They ignited my interest in health law and have provided daily counsel on a variety of professional and personal matters over the years. I earnestly hope that as my daughter proceeds through school and her professional life, she is fortunate enough to have such capable, patient, and caring mentors.

I am also thankful to Eric Gordon, Robert Jensen, Robert Louthian, Jim Sneed, and Eric Zimmerman for their editorial comments and invaluable suggestions as to how to improve this work. Dariel Hendy provided indispensible support in revising and proofing numerous edits of this work.

Most of all, I wish to thank my wife, Toinette. Writing this book occupied most weekends and many evenings for over a year. During this time, Toinette was pregnant with and gave birth to our first child, Madeline Grace Reynolds. Nonetheless, Toinette liberated me to fulfill my long-time professional ambition to write this book.

About the Author

Max M. Reynolds is a partner in the Health Law Department of McDermott, Will & Emery's Washington, D.C. office. He regularly counsels acute care hospitals, physicians, clinical laboratories, and other health care providers on regulatory issues, including Medicare reimbursement and fraud and abuse compliance matters.

Mr. Reynolds has published extensively on Medicare regulatory matters as well as on health care fraud and abuse. His work includes articles on EMTALA, the hospital outpatient prospective payment system, the hospital inpatient prospective payment system, the rehabilitation facility prospective payment system, and gainsharing. The articles include "Gainsharing: A Cost-Reduction Strategy that May Be Back" in the January 2002 issue of *Healthcare Financial Management;* "Final Inpatient Rehabilitation PPS Rule Improves on Proposed Rule," in the October 2001 *Healthcare Financial Management;* "EMTALA Liability: Transforming Your Off-Campus Facility into an Emergency Department," in the January 2001 *Trustee;* "Medicare Payment for New Impatient Services and Technologies Requires Expanded Coordination Between Hospitals and Those Conducting Clinical Trials," in *The RAP Sheet*, Summer 2001; and "HCFA's New Restrictions on the Operation of Hospital Outpatient Facilities," in the *Journal of Health Law*, Fall 2000.

Mr. Reynolds received a bachelor's degree in political science, *summa cum laude* and Phi Beta Kappa, from Emory University in 1992. He earned a J.D. in 1996 from the University of Virginia. He is admitted to practice in the District of Columbia and the Commonwealth of Virginia.

CHAPTER 1

Overview

Hospitals are forming joint ventures with staff physicians and others in increasing numbers. Hospitals have seized on joint ventures as a reliable mechanism to promote physician loyalty, attract and retain clinical expertise, defray costs associated with capital-intensive projects, and negotiate with third-party payers. Such joint venture arrangements must be structured carefully, however, in order to ensure compliance with a broad array of federal and state laws.

THE GROWTH OF HOSPITAL JOINT VENTURES

There is general consensus that the number and array of joint ventures involving hospitals has grown significantly in recent years. Many such joint ventures involving hospitals are clinical in nature; that is, they are formed to acquire and operate general acute care hospitals, specialty hospitals, subacute providers, surgical facilities, diagnostic imaging centers, clinics, or other facilities in which patient care is furnished. Other joint ventures serve a support function, as in physician–hospital organizations formed to contract with managed care organizations, and management companies formed to acquire and lease office space to members of a hospital's medical staff.

Hospitals recognize a number of benefits associated with joint venture arrangements. First, when the joint venture involves members of the hospital's medical staff, the arrangement might foster physician loyalty and/or preempt physicians from independently offering lucrative services in competition with the hospital. This, too, is a particularly important consideration, given that the common hospital-physician bonding devices employed throughout the 1990s have proven financially infeasible (such as in physician practice acquisitions), administratively infeasible (such as in many types of physician–hospital integrated delivery systems), or to be of questionable legality (as in gainsharing). Second, hospitals can use the option of equity investment to attract and retain individuals with the requisite administrative or clinical expertise to ensure cost-effective operations. Third, joint ventures enable hospitals to share the cost associated with capital-intensive undertakings. This is a significant advantage, given the high cost of clinical facilities and platforms at a time when approximately one-third of all hospitals maintain a negative operating margin. Finally, well-designed integrated delivery system joint ventures might enable hospitals to extract more lucrative compensation from third-party payers.

AN OVERVIEW OF THIS HANDBOOK

Although hospital joint ventures offer these and other benefits, they can, unless properly structured, pose significant legal risks under federal and state laws. These risks include those relating to health care fraud and abuse, restrictions on joint venture activity by tax-exempt institutions, antitrust restrictions, and the issuance of securities. Moreover, numerous agencies within the federal government have recently announced their intention to scrutinize hospital joint venture arrangements more closely. For example, the Department of Health and Human Services Office of Inspector General released a Special Advisory Bulletin in April 2003 describing characteristics of abusive hospital joint venture arrangements and announcing its intent to target those participating in them. Additionally, during the late summer of 2003, the Federal Trade Commission and the Department of Justice have jointly held an unprecedented series of hearings on anticompetitive practices in the health care industry and specifically addressed anticompetitiveness concerns associated with hospital joint ventures.

In light of the growing reliance by hospitals on joint ventures with staff physicians and the clear intent of the federal government to scrutinize such arrangements more heavily than ever, hospital executives will need a resource that (1) summarizes the pertinent federal laws potentially implicated by hospital joint ventures, (2) identifies the risks that joint venture activity poses under these laws, and (3) suggests strategies by which hospital executives can structure and operate joint ventures that meet their business objectives while minimizing compliance concerns.

This handbook is written to address that need. It focuses upon the unique federal regulatory considerations that must be addressed in any hospital joint venture arrangement. These include health care fraud and abuse law, tax law, antitrust law, securities law, and Medicare certification and enrollment. A hospital joint venture might involve other federal laws in the ordinary course of business that are not unique to the joint venture setting, for example, requirements governing occupational safety, disposal of radioactive materials, confidentiality of patient information. Also, numerous state laws of all types might be involved. However, such compliance concerns are not addressed herein. Rather this work will focus specifically upon those federal laws raising unique concerns in the joint venture context.

The first part of this handbook includes separate chapters describing federal laws relating to health care fraud and abuse, tax, antitrust, securities, and Medicare certification and enrollment, assessing how they are implicated by hospital joint ventures, and analyzing how hospitals and fellow joint venture participants can facilitate compliance with these laws. The second part of the work includes separate chapters describing the regulatory implications and compliance strategies associated with various aspects of the joint venture arrangement, namely investor selection, structuring the joint venture, and operating the joint venture on an ongoing basis.

CHAPTER 2

Federal Fraud and Abuse Laws Governing Hospital Joint Ventures

INTRODUCTION

Special care must be taken to ensure that joint ventures are structured and operated in compliance with applicable federal health care program ("Federal Program") fraud and abuse laws.[1] The Department of Health and Human Services Office of Inspector General ("OIG"), the Centers for Medicare and Medicaid Services ("CMS") and the Department of Justice ("DOJ") have scrutinized joint venture arrangements in recent years to ensure compliance with Federal Program integrity requirements. They have focused principally upon compliance with three distinct federal laws: the federal health care program anti-kickback law ("Anti-Kickback Law"), the federal physician self-referral law ("Stark Law"), and the federal health care program exclusion law ("Exclusion Law").[2] The provisions of, and compliance concerns associated with, each statute are addressed below.

ANTI-KICKBACK LAW

General Provisions

The Anti-Kickback Law generally prohibits any person from "knowingly and willfully" offering or paying "remuneration" to "induce" another to (1) refer patients for the provision of items or services that may be paid for by a Federal Program, (2) purchase, lease, or order such items or services, or (3) recommend or arrange for the purchase, lease, or order of such items or services.[3] The Anti-Kickback Law also prohibits the knowing and willful solicitation or acceptance of such remuneration.[4]

The OIG defines the term "remuneration" broadly to cover "anything of value."[5] The term "inducement" also has been interpreted broadly to cover any act that is intended to "influence" the "reason or judgment of another in an effort to cause the referral of program-related business."[6] Further, the fact that there are legitimate reasons for the remuneration at issue is irrelevant; the OIG and federal courts have taken the position that so long as "one of the purposes" of the payment is to induce the referral of Federal Program business, the Anti-Kickback Law is implicated.[7]

Violation of the Anti-Kickback Law is punishable by criminal or civil sanctions. Criminal sanctions include five years imprisonment, a $25,000 fine, and mandatory exclusion from participation in Federal Programs.[8] Civil sanctions include a $50,000 civil money penalty, an assessment of up to three times the amount of remuneration involved, and potential exclusion from all Federal Programs.[9]

Recognizing that the Anti-Kickback Law is "extremely broad" and that "many relatively innocuous or even beneficial commercial arrangements are technically covered by the statute and are therefore subject to criminal prosecution," Congress has enacted a number of statutory "exceptions"—and the OIG has promulgated a number of regulatory "safe harbors"—protecting certain arrangements involving a low risk of fraud and abuse.[10] In order to qualify for protection, however, an arrangement must precisely meet each of the requirements in an exception or safe harbor; substantial compliance will not suffice.[11] Failure to comply with an exception or safe harbor, however, "does not make an arrangement per se illegal."[12] Rather, the OIG will scrutinize the arrangement on a "case-by-case basis" to assess the "potential risk of fraud and abuse."[13] Factors pertinent to this assessment most likely include the effect of the arrangement on the following: access to health care services, quality of care, patient freedom of choice among providers, competition among providers, costs to Federal Programs, the potential for overutilization, and the ability of health care facilities to provide services in medically underserved areas or to medically underserved populations.[14] If parties are uncertain as to how the OIG might view an arrangement, they can request an advisory opinion from the OIG.[15]

Application to Hospital Joint Ventures

The OIG's principal concern when evaluating joint venture arrangements under the Anti-Kickback Law is whether the venture's investment distributions and operating arrangements (e.g., leases, employment agreements, personal services agreements, sales contracts, loans) include or constitute disguised payment (i.e., "remuneration") for: (1) the referral of Federal Program patients to the joint venture or between fellow investors outside the joint venture framework, (2) the purchase, lease, or order of items or services from the joint venture or its investors which may be paid for by a Federal Program, or (3) recommending or arranging for the purchase, lease, or order of items or services from the joint venture or its investors that may be paid for by a Federal Program.[16]

Consequently, the OIG focuses on joint venture arrangements in which investors and others receiving compensation are in a position to generate Federal Program business for the venture or fellow investors.[17] The OIG has repeatedly noted that the foregoing concerns are not limited to situations in which physicians receive joint venture distributions or payments. Rather, fraud and abuse concerns also arise when hospitals receive such distributions or payments because they too are able to steer Federal Program business.[18]

Joint Venture Investment Distributions

Joint venture investment distributions and operating agreements raise similar but somewhat distinct compliance concerns under the Anti-Kickback, and are therefore addressed separately below.

As noted above, the government will scrutinize joint venture investment distributions to determine whether they equate a commercially reasonable return on investment for capital placed at genuine risk or, alternatively, include or constitute disguised payment for the referral of Federal Program business by hospital or physician investors. In the joint venture illustrated in the diagram, the government will scrutinize the following:

- Was joint venture equity participation offered to the selected physicians as a means of rewarding past referrals and/or inducing future referrals to the joint venture or to the offered investing hospital outside the joint venture?

- Was joint venture equity participation to the hospital as a means of rewarding and/or inducing the hospital to, in turn, encourage its employed physicians, contractor physicians, or staff physicians to refer patients to the joint venture or to the physician investors in connection with their clinical practices outside the joint venture?

Joint Venture Investment Distributions

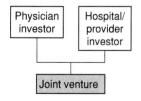

Safe Harbor Protection. Parties to a joint venture can eliminate the risk of liability under the Anti-Kickback Law from receipt of joint venture distributions by structuring the joint venture in strict compliance with the terms of the safe harbor for general investment interests or the safe harbor for ambulatory surgical center investment interests. The provisions of each safe harbor are described below.

Investment Interests Safe Harbor

The most broadly applicable safe-harbor-protecting joint venture distributions is the "Investment Interests Safe Harbor."[19] The safe harbor is predicated upon the OIG's belief that investment distributions are more likely to constitute a legitimate return for capital placed at genuine risk (rather than an impermissible inducement for the generation or referral of Federal Program business) when the joint venture (1) raises substantial capital from individuals who do not generate business for the joint venture, (2) does not rely principally upon business from investors, (3) does not require investors to generate business, and (4) makes distributions to investors only in proportion to the amount of capital they have genuinely placed at risk in the venture.[20] The provisions in "Investment Interests Safe Harbor" specifically protect any dividend or other "return on investment" paid by the joint venture to an investor so long as each of the following requirements are met:

- **Substantial Base of Nonbusiness Source Investors:** No more than 40% of the value of each class of investment interests in the joint venture was held in the previous fiscal year or previous 12-month period by investors who were in a position to make or influence referrals to, furnish items or services to, or otherwise generate business for the joint venture ("Potential Business Source Investors").[21] (This provision is designed to ensure that safe harbor protection is afforded only (1) to those joint ventures that are capable of securing capital from independent sources who will not generate business for or from the joint venture and (2) when any joint venture profit distributions will be made "to a wider group" than those generating business for the joint venture.[22] For purposes of this requirement, investment interests held by an entity will be deemed to be held by the entity and imputed proportionally to its investors and beyond until all interests are allotted to individuals).[23]

- **Consistent Investment Terms for Business-Source and Nonbusiness-Source Passive Investors:** The terms on which an investment interest is offered to a passive investor, if any, who is a Potential Business Source Investor must be no different from the terms offered to other passive investors.[24] (This provision is designed to preclude protection for joint venture arrangements involving "discriminatory marketing strategies that result in the offer of better deals" to Potential Business Source Passive Investors rather than Nonbusiness Source Passive Investors).[25]

- **Independently Determined Investment Terms for Potential Business-Source Investors:** The terms on which an investment interest is offered to an investor who is a Potential Business Source Investor must not be related to the previous or expected volume of referrals, items or services furnished, or other business generated from that investor to the joint venture.[26] (This provision "assumes that an investment interest is being offered to a person in a position to make referrals" or generate business for the joint venture, but "bars the offering of favorable terms based upon [the investor's] past or expected referrals" to the joint venture or the past or expected volume of items or services furnished or business generated for the joint venture).[27]

- **Protecting Those Who Are/Become Nonbusiness Source Investors:** There is no requirement that a passive investor, if any, make referrals to, be in a position to make or influence referrals to, furnish items or services to, or otherwise generate business for the joint venture as a condition for remaining as an investor.[28] (This provision precludes safe harbor protection for arrangements in which an investor is divested of his or her investment interest if he or she fails to generate sufficient business for the joint venture).[29]

- **Nondiscrimination Among Passive Investors:** Neither the joint venture nor any joint venture investor markets or furnishes the joint venture's items or services (or those of another joint venture as part of a cross-referral agreement) to passive investors differently than to noninvestors.[30]

- **Substantial Base of Joint Venture Business from Noninvestors:** No more than 40% of the joint venture's gross revenue related to the furnishing of health care items and services in the previous fiscal year or previous 12-month period came from referrals or business otherwise generated from investors.[31] (This provision is designed to ensure that safe harbor protection is (1) not afforded to joint ventures "that operate primarily on the referrals of" investors and (2) afforded only where joint venture profit distributions will be distributed "to a wider group than referring physician investors."[32] For purposes of this requirement, investment interests held by an entity will be deemed to be held by the entity and imputed proportionally to its investors and beyond until all interests are allotted to individuals).[33]

- **No Loans to Business Source Investors to Acquire Their Investment Interest:** Neither the joint venture nor any investor (nor anyone acting on their behalf) loans funds to or guarantees a loan for a Potential Business Source Investor if the investor uses any part of such loan to obtain the investment interest.[34] (This provision is designed to ensure that an investor's funds are "genuinely at risk" in the joint venture, that is, to "assure that physicians and other investors in fact provide new needed capital and that the joint venture is not in reality a sham to facilitate the distribution of payments for referrals."[35])

- **Investment Returns Proportionate to Invested Capital:** The investment returns paid to each investor are proportionate to the amount of his or her capital investment (including the fair market value of any pre-operational services rendered).[36]

For purposes of the safe harbor, an "investor" is any individual or entity who holds a direct or indirect investment interest in the joint venture. An indirect interest may arise when one: (1) obtains a beneficial interest in the joint venture (for example, beneficiary status in a trust holding an interest in the joint venture), (2) uses an intermediary to hold an interest in the joint venture, or (3) maintains an ownership interest in an entity which, in turn, invests in the joint venture.[37] An "active investor" is one who (1) is a general partner in the joint venture and is "responsible for the day-to-day management" of the venture or (2) agrees in writing to undertake liability for the actions of the joint venture's agents acting within the scope of their duties.[38] All other investors are "passive investors" for purposes of the safe harbor.[39]

ASC Safe Harbor

If a joint venture is limited to the establishment and operation of an ambulatory surgical center ("ASC"), any dividend or other "return on investment" paid by the joint venture to an investor may be protected under the Investment Interests Safe Harbor (described above) or a specific safe harbor for ASC joint ventures (the "ASC Safe Harbor").[40]

The OIG's "chief concern" regarding distributions to investors in an ASC joint venture, as with distributions from other types of joint ventures, is that "a return on an investment in an ASC might be disguised payment" for Federal Program referrals or other Federal Program business.[41] For example, a primary care physician might be offered an investment interest in an ASC "as an incentive to refer patients to the surgeon owners of the ASC."[42] The OIG concludes that this risk is substantially reduced when the physician investor's practice is so integrated with the ASC that the facility serves as an "extension of the physician's office practice."[43] "Where the ASC is functionally an extension of a physician's office, so that the physician personally performs services at the ASC on his or her own patients as a substantial part of his or her medical practice, we believe that the ASC serves a bona fide business purpose and that the risk of improper payments for referrals is relatively low."[44]

To date, the OIG has not been willing to extend safe harbor protection to other types of ancillary services joint ventures on this alternative basis. The additional and unique avenue for safe harbor protection of ASC joint ventures "derives in large measure" from (1) the government's "longstanding policy encouraging freestanding ASCs as a less costly alternative to hospitals for appropriate surgeries" and (2) the fact that Medicare reimbursement for an ASC procedure is dictated by a "prospectively established ASC payment methodology."[45]

The ASC Safe Harbor specifically protects any dividend or other "return on investment" paid by an ASC joint venture to an investor so long as each of the following requirements is met:

- The ASC is certified by Medicare.[46]

- The ASC has exclusive use of its operating room and recovery room space.[47] (This space cannot be shared with the hospital for the use of its registered inpatients and outpatients.[48] This safeguard is designed to ensure that the hospital does not obtain indirect reimbursement through its cost report for expenses incurred in connection with the ASC joint venture.)

- Patients referred to the ASC joint venture by investors "are fully informed of the investor's investment interest."[49] (According to the OIG, this provision is designed to protect "patient freedom of choice" and "informed decision making, though it does not—in isolation—provide sufficient assurance against fraud and abuse."[50])

- The terms on which an investment interest in the ASC joint venture is offered to an investor are not related to the previous or expected volume of referrals, services furnished, or the amount of business otherwise generated from the investor to the ASC.[51]

- Neither the ASC joint venture nor any joint venture investor (nor any person acting on their behalf) loans funds to or guarantees a loan for a fellow investor for acquisition of an interest in the joint venture.[52]

- The amount of payment to an investor in return for his or her investment in the ASC joint venture is directly proportional to the amount of his or her capital investment (including the fair market value of any pre-operational services rendered).[53]

- The ASC joint venture and any hospital or physician investor treats Federal Program beneficiaries in a nondiscriminatory manner.[54]

- The ASC joint venture does not use space (including, but not limited to, operating and recovery room space) located in or owned by any hospital investor, unless such space is leased from the hospital in accordance with a lease that complies with all the standards of the Anti-Kickback Law space rental safe harbor.[55]

- The ASC joint venture does not use equipment owned by any hospital investor, unless such equipment is leased in accordance with a lease that complies with the Anti-Kickback Law equipment rental safe harbor.[56]

- The ASC joint venture does not use services provided by a hospital investor, unless such services are provided in accordance with a contract that complies with the Anti-Kickback Law personal services and management contracts safe harbor.[57]

- All ancillary services for Federal Program beneficiaries performed at the joint venture ASC are "directly and integrally related" to "primary" procedures performed at the ASC, and none are separately billed to Federal Programs.[58]

- The hospital investor does not include any costs associated with the joint venture ASC on its cost report or any claim for payment from a Federal Program (unless specifically required to do so by law).[59]

- The hospital is not in a position to make or influence referrals directly or indirectly to any investor or the ASC joint venture.[60] (A hospital will generally be deemed a referral source for an ASC joint venture so as to preclude safe harbor protection.[61] Nonetheless, OIG advisory opinions suggest that arrangements that otherwise meet the ASC Safe Harbor requirements will pose minimal risk of fraud and abuse if appropriate measures are taken to constrain the hospital's ability to refer patients to the ASC joint venture. Safeguards would include: (1) the hospital refraining from encouraging employed, contractor, or staff physicians to refer patients to the joint venture ASC or joint venture investors, (2) refraining from tracking referrals from these physicians to the joint venture ASC or joint venture investors, (3) refraining from directly or indirectly predicating compensation to these physicians on referrals to the joint venture ASC or ASC investors, and (4) informing these physicians of the foregoing policies at least annually.[62])

- The nonhospital ASC joint venture investors who are employed by the joint venture or any joint venture investor or are otherwise in a position to refer patients or furnish items or services to the joint venture or joint venture investors collectively fall into one of the following categories:[63]

  - They are all general surgeons, group practices of general surgeons, surgeons of the same specialty, or group practices of the same specialty and one-third of each surgeon investor's "medical practice income" from all sources in the prior fiscal year or 12 months was derived from ASC-Approved Procedures.[64]

  - They are all physicians in the same "medical practice specialty" or groups of physicians in the same medical practice specialty, and one-third of each physician investor's "medical practice income" from all sources in the prior fiscal year or 12 months was derived from ASC-Approved Procedures.[65]

  - They are all physicians in a position to refer patients to the ASC joint venture and perform procedures on such referred patients (or group practices composed of such physicians) and both of the following conditions are met: (1) one-third of each physician investor's "medical practice income" from all sources in the prior fiscal year or 12 months was derived from ASC-Approved Procedures and (2) one-third of the ASC-Approved Procedures performed by each physician investor in the previous fiscal year or previous 12 months was performed at the ASC joint venture.[66]

For purposes of the ASC Safe Harbor, the term "ASC-Approved Procedures" refers to those procedures authorized by Medicare for reimbursement in an ASC setting, *even if* such procedures were performed in a hospital setting.[67] The term "group practice" has the same meaning as under the Stark Law, described below.[68] Finally, an ASC joint venture interest held by a physician's professional corporation is deemed to be held directly by the physician for purposes of the ASC Safe Harbor.[69]

Risk Analysis. If joint venture distributions do not qualify for protection under one of the foregoing safe harbors, they will not necessarily violate the Anti-Kickback Law. Rather, the OIG will scrutinize the manner in which joint venture investors are selected and the joint venture is operated in order to assess the degree of risk that joint venture distributions include or constitute impermissible remuneration under the Anti-Kickback Law.[70] In subsequent chapters, we describe how hospital joint venture arrangements can be structured so as to minimize the fraud and abuse risks on each count.[71]

Joint Venture Operating Arrangements. Even if joint venture investment distributions are protected by one of the foregoing safe harbors, vetted in a favorable OIG advisory opinion, or otherwise structured in a manner which minimizes the risk of Federal Program abuse, the OIG's concern with the joint venture will not be altogether eliminated. Rather, the OIG will also scrutinize operating arrangements (such as leases, employment agreements, personal services agreements, sales contracts, and loans) between the joint venture and investors or other third parties who are in a position to refer Federal Program beneficiaries to, furnish Federal Program items or services to, or otherwise generate Federal Program business for the joint venture or fellow investors. Specifically, the OIG will inquire whether payments made pursuant to such operating arrangements constitute commercially reasonable consideration for items or services furnished or, alternatively, contain remuneration for the referral or generation of Federal Program Business for the joint venture or one or more of its investors.[72]

Safe Harbor Protection. Parties to an operating agreement can eliminate the risk of liability under the Anti-Kickback Law in connection with payments by the joint venture by structuring the arrangement in strict compliance with the terms of a pertinent safe harbor. The three principal safe harbors for operating arrangements are Lease Safe Harbor, Employee Safe Harbor, and Personal Services Safe Harbor. Each of these is described in the sections that follow.

Lease Safe Harbor

Rental payments for equipment, realty, or personalty are protected under the Lease Safe Harbor so long as each of the following requirements is met:

- The lease is set out in writing and signed by the parties.[73]

- The lease covers all of the premises or equipment leased between the parties for the term of the lease and specifies the premises or equipment covered by the lease.[74]

- If the lease is intended to provide the lessee with access to the premises or equipment for periodic intervals of time, rather than on a full-time basis for the term of the lease, the lease specifies the schedule of such intervals, their precise length, and the exact rent for such intervals.[75] (This provision is designed to ensure that the parties do not vary the frequency or duration of lease intervals with the volume or value of Federal Program business).[76]

- The term of the lease is for not less than one year.[77] (This provision is designed to preclude safe harbor protection where parties frequently renegotiate compensation terms for short-term agreements to reflect the volume or value of Federal Program business generated between them.[78] An agreement may include a for-cause termination provision and still qualify for safe harbor status so long as the agreement provides that, upon termination, the parties will not renegotiate the contract or engage in further commercial arrangements during the remaining one-year term of the initial arrangement.[79])

- The aggregate rental charge is set in advance, is consistent with fair market value in arms-length transactions and is not determined in a manner that takes into account the volume or value of any referrals or business otherwise generated between the parties for which payment may be made in whole or in part by a Federal Program.[80] (Fixed per-use or per-unit-of-service fees do not receive safe harbor protection because they (1) are not fixed in "aggregate" and (2) may vary with the volume or value of referrals. Rather, the OIG reviews such arrangements on a case-by-case basis to assess the potential for fraud and abuse).[81]

- The aggregate space or equipment rented does not exceed that which is reasonably necessary to accomplish the commercially reasonable business purpose of the rental.[82] (The OIG states that this provision "is intended to preclude safe harbor protection for health care providers that surreptitiously pay for referrals—whether because of coercion or by their own initiative—by renting more space or equipment or purchasing more services than they actually need from referral sources."[83])

When the Lease Safe Harbor is invoked in connection with rental of space, the term "fair market value" means the value of the rental property for general commercial purposes, but shall not be adjusted to reflect the additional value that one party (either the prospective lessee or lessor) would attribute to the property as a result of its proximity or convenience to sources of referrals or other business for which payment may be made in whole or in part by a Federal Program.[84] When the Lease Safe Harbor is invoked in connection with rental of equipment, the term "fair market value" means the value of the equipment when obtained from a manufacturer or professional distributor, but shall not be adjusted to reflect the additional value one party (either the prospective lessee or lessor) would attribute to the equipment as a result of its proximity or convenience to sources of referrals or other business for which payment may be made in whole or in part by a Federal Program.[85]

Employee Safe Harbor

The Employee Safe Harbor is quite broad, protecting payments by an "employer" to a bona fide "employee" for employment in the furnishing of items or services.[86] Although the safe harbor does not include an explicit requirement that payments made to an employee be equivalent to fair market value for services actually furnished to the employer, failure to adhere to such a standard will increase the risk that the OIG will deem payments to an employee to be for something other than the furnishing of items or services on behalf of the employer and, therefore, beyond the protection of the Employee Safe Harbor.

Personal Services Safe Harbor

Payments made for personal services furnished by nonemployees ("agents") will be protected under the Personal Services Safe Harbor so long as each of the following requirements is met:

- The agreement is set out in writing and signed by the parties.[87]

- The agreement covers all of the services the agent provides to the principal for the term of the agreement and specifies the services to be provided by the agent.[88]

- If the agreement is intended to provide for the services of the agent on a periodic, sporadic or part-time basis, rather than on a full-time basis for the term of the agreement, the agreement specifies the schedule of such intervals, their precise duration, and the exact charge for such intervals.[89] (This provision is designed to ensure that the parties do not vary the frequency or duration of service intervals with the volume or value of Federal Program business.[90])

- The term of the agreement is for not less than one year.[91] (This provision is designed to preclude safe harbor protection where parties frequently renegotiate compensation terms for short-term agreements to reflect the volume or value of Federal Program business generated between them.[92] An agreement may include a for-cause termination provision and still qualify for safe harbor status so long as the agreement provides that, upon termination, the parties will not renegotiate the contract or engage in further commercial arrangements during the remaining one-year term of the initial arrangement.[93])

- The aggregate compensation paid to the agent over the term of the agreement is set in advance, is consistent with fair market value in arms-length transactions and is not determined in a manner that takes into account the volume or value of any referrals or business otherwise generated between the parties for which payment may be made in whole or in part under Federal Programs.[94] (Fixed per-use or per-unit-of-service fees do not receive safe harbor protection as they (1) are not fixed in "aggregate" and (2) may vary with the volume or value of referrals.[95] Rather, the OIG reviews such arrangements on a case-by-case basis to assess the potential for fraud and abuse.[96])

- The aggregate services contracted for do not exceed those that are reasonably necessary to accomplish the commercially reasonable business purpose of the services.[97] (The OIG states that this provision "is intended to preclude safe harbor protection for health care providers that surreptitiously pay for referrals—whether because of coercion or by their own initiative—by renting more space or equipment or purchasing more services than they actually need from referral sources."[98])

- The services performed under the agreement do not involve the counseling or promotion of a business arrangement or other activity that violates any state or federal law.[99]

Risk Analysis. If joint venture operating agreements do not qualify for protection under one of the foregoing safe harbors, they will not necessarily violate the Anti-Kickback Law. Rather, the OIG will scrutinize the agreement on a case-by-case basis to determine whether payments pursuant to the agreement include or constitute impermissible remuneration under the Anti-Kickback Law.[100] The OIG's concern that an operating arrangement includes impermissible remuneration will be minimized where the arrangement is memorialized and contains only commercially reasonable terms (i.e., terms similar to those which would be negotiated by parties who do not generate business for each other and are acting at arm's length).[101] In Chapter 9, we describe how such arrangements can be structured so as to minimize the fraud and abuse risks on each count.

THE STARK LAW

General Provisions

The Stark Law reflects concern that a physician with a financial stake in determining whether or where to make a referral may be "unduly influenced by a profit motive," and thereby inclined to overutilize items or services paid for by the federal government or "steer" patients to "less convenient, lower quality, or more expensive providers of health care."[102]

The Law generally prohibits a physician from referring Medicare beneficiaries to an entity for the furnishing of designated health services ("DHS") if the physician has a nonexempt "financial relationship" with the entity.[103] DHS include:

- Inpatient and outpatient hospital services.
- Clinical laboratory services.
- Physical and occupational therapy.
- Speech-language pathology.
- Radiology and certain other imaging services.
- Radiation therapy services and supplies.
- Durable medical equipment and supplies.
- Home health services.
- Outpatient prescription drugs.
- Prosthetics and orthotics.
- Parenteral and enteral nutrients, equipment, and supplies.[104]

The term "referral" is defined broadly to include any request for, ordering of, or certifying of the need for (1) DHS or (2) a consultation that results in the furnishing of DHS, unless the physician ostensibly "referring" the patient "personally" furnishes the DHS (i.e., the physician physically performs the DHS himself or herself without reliance on other clinical staff or physicians).[105] The following unique rules apply to requests for clinical laboratory services, radiology services, and radiation therapy services:

- When a physician requests a consultation by a pathologist and such pathologist orders clinical diagnostic testing services, the physician requesting the consultation is deemed to have made the referral for the diagnostic tests.[106] (The pathologist may also be deemed to have made a referral for the service unless he or she furnishes or supervises performance of the tests).

- When a physician requests a consultation from a radiologist who orders diagnostic radiology services, the physician requesting the consultation will be deemed to have made the referral for the service.[107] (The radiologist may also be deemed to have made a referred for the services unless he or she furnishes or supervises performance of the radiology services).

- When a physician requests a consultation from a radiation oncologist who orders radiation therapy, the physician requesting the consultation will be deemed to have made the referral for the radiology or radiation therapy service.[108] (The radiation oncologist may also be deemed to have made a referral for the service unless he or she furnishes or supervises performance of the radiation therapy).

The Stark Law also prohibits any entity from billing Medicare for DHS furnished pursuant to a prohibited referral.[109] Any payments (including copayments) received in violation of this prohibition must be promptly refunded.[110] Unless such refund is made on a timely basis, the Department of Health and Human Services ("HHS") may impose a civil money penalty of up to $15,000 against any person who (1) presented or caused presentation of the claim and (2) knew or should have known the claim resulted from an impermissible referral.[111] Such persons may also be excluded from participation in Federal Programs.[112] Congress and CMS have, however, provided several discrete exceptions to the referral and billing prohibition. Pertinent exceptions are described below.

Application to Hospital Joint Ventures

If a joint venture furnishes DHS, representatives must ensure that the venture (1) is financed and operated in a manner that precludes creation of nonexempt financial relationships with referring physicians and (2) does not bill Medicare, absent an applicable Stark Law exception, for DHS furnished pursuant to a referral from a physician with whom it has a nonexempt financial relationship. Whether or not it furnishes DHS, the joint venture might consider—as a prudential matter rather than a legal obligation—apprising potential investors if participation in the arrangement might give rise to an indirect financial relationship between the physician and the joint venture or some other entity that furnishes DHS to Medicare beneficiaries.

Next we summarize the principal scenarios in which a physician investing in the joint venture might incur a nonexempt financial relationship with an entity furnishing DHS and describe the circumstances under which DHS furnished to a Medicare beneficiary pursuant to such a referral might nonetheless be billed to the Medicare program. In succeeding chapters, we will describe steps that joint venture representatives can take to minimize Stark Law liability for the joint venture and its investors.[113]

Financial Relationships Involving Joint Venture Investors

Unless appropriate safeguards are observed, a joint venture arrangement might create a financial relationship generally precluding a physician investor from referring Medicare patients to the joint venture as well as certain health care providers compensating the joint venture.

Investor Referrals to the Joint Venture

Physicians investing in a joint venture through equity or secured debt will incur a "financial relationship" with the joint venture in the form of an "ownership or investment interest."[114] This financial relationship arises regardless of whether the physician maintains his or her interest directly (i.e., personally holds an investment interest in the joint venture as depicted in the upper-left part of the diagram) or indirectly (i.e., there is a chain of one or more juridical entities or intermediaries between the physician and the joint venture, and each successive entity between the physician and the joint venture holds an investment interest in the entity below it, as depicted in the upper-right part of the diagram).[115] Consequently, under either circumstance, the investor physicians will be precluded from referring Medicare beneficiaries to the joint venture for DHS, and the joint venture will be prohibited from billing Medicare for DHS furnished pursuant to such a referral, assuming it acts in reckless disregard of the physician's investment interest, unless one of the following exceptions applies:

- **Personally Furnished Services.** The investing physician personally furnishes any DHS provided to the patient at the joint venture (i.e., the physician physically performs the service and does not rely on other physicians or clinical staff).[116]

- **Qualified DHS.** The DHS furnished to the Medicare beneficiary is limited to the following types of DHS ("Qualified DHS"):

Investor Referrals to the Joint Venture

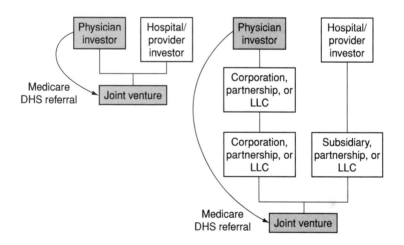

- Clinical laboratory services furnished in an ASC, ESRD facility, or hospice and included in the ASC rate, ESRD composite rate, or the per-diem hospice charge.[117]

- Designated dialysis-related outpatient prescription drugs administered or dispensed by an ESRD facility.[118]

- Designated preventive screening tests, immunizations, and vaccines.[119]

- Eyeglasses and contact lenses covered by Medicare when furnished to patients following cataract surgery.[120]

- Implants (including, without limitation, cochlear implants, intraocular lenses, implanted prosthetic devices, and implanted DME) furnished by the referring physician or a member of his or her group practice and implanted in a surgical procedure performed at the certified ASC where the implant is furnished.[121]

- **Qualified Prepaid Health Plan Services.** The Medicare beneficiary is enrolled in a qualified "prepaid health plan."[122] Qualified prepaid plans include the following: (1) certain health plans that contract with CMS pursuant to § 1876 of the Social Security Act, (2) a health care prepayment plan that contracts with CMS pursuant to § 1833(a)(1)(A) of the Social Security Act, (3) health plans receiving payment on a prepaid basis pursuant to certain demonstration projects authorized under the Social Security Act, (4) a health maintenance organization ("HMO") qualified under the Federal HMO Act, or (5) a Medicare+Choice coordinated care plan.[123]

- **Whole-Hospital Exception.** The joint venture is a hospital at which the investing physician maintains staff privileges, and the investing physician's investment interest is in the entire hospital rather than a mere subdivision or department of the facility.[124] (Please note that § 507 of P.L. 108-___ makes this exception unavailable until May 18, 2005 for "specialty hospitals" outside of Puerto Rico unless they were in operation nor under development as of November 18, 2003 and have not done any of the following since that date: (1) increased the number of physician investors, (2) added certain categories of new clinical services, (3) added bed capacity in contravention of certain restrictions, or (4) violates other requirements to be designated by the Secretary. For purposes of this restriction, a "specialty hospital" is one "primarily or exclusively" engaged in treating patients with a cardiac or orthopedic condition, undergoing surgery, or receiving any other "specialized category of services" that the Secretary designates as "inconsistent with the purpose of permitting physician ownership and investment interests in a hospital" under the "Whole Hospital Investment Interest Exception.")

- **Qualified Rural Clinical Services.** The joint venture furnishes DHS to the patient in a rural area and "substantially all" of its DHS is furnished to residents of a rural area.[125]

- **Qualified Group Practice Services.** The joint venture is a physician "group practice," the DHS furnished qualifies as a "physician service," and the physician furnishing the service is an equity owner in, an employee of, or contractor for the group ("Group Practice Exception").[126] A joint venture will only qualify as a "group" practice if each of the following requirements is satisfied:

  - The joint venture is a "single legal entity formed primarily for the purpose of being a group practice" and is not organized or owned (in whole or part) by another medical practice.

  - The joint venture has at least two physicians as shareholders or employees.

  - Each physician shareholder and physician employee uses the joint venture's shared office space, equipment, and personnel to furnish "substantially the full range" of the "patient care services" he or she "routinely performs".

  - 75% of the aggregate of all "patient care services" of the joint venture's physician shareholders and physician employees are furnished by the joint venture and billed under the joint venture's billing number.

  - The joint venture's overhead and income are distributed according to methods determined before receipt of payment for the services giving rise to such overhead or income.

  - The joint venture is a "unified business" with centralized decision-making and utilization review as well as consolidated billing, accounting, and financial reporting.

  - Physician shareholders and employees do not receive compensation based on the volume or value of DHS referrals they make other than through qualified productivity bonuses or profit shares.

  - Physician shareholders or employees perform at least 75% of the joint venture's patient–physician encounters.[127]

  Additionally, applicable state law must permit the entity to qualify as a "group" practice even though one or more shareholder members are not physicians.[128]

- **Qualified In-Office Ancillary Services.** The joint venture is a physician "group practice,"[129] and the DHS furnished qualifies as an "in-office ancillary service" by satisfying the following requirements ("In-Office Ancillary Services Exception"):

- Receipt of DHS is not the "primary" reason the patient comes in contact with the referring physician.[130]

- The DHS is furnished with the level of physician supervision required by Medicare regulations (i.e., general, direct, or personal), and the physician responsible for such supervision is (1) a shareholder in the Group, (2) an employee of the Group, or (3) an independent contractor.[131]

- The DHS is furnished either in a space used exclusively by the group in a centralized building for the furnishing of DHS or, alternatively, at a location at which the group maintains an office housing at least one physician employee or physician shareholder who provides substantial physician services unrelated to the furnishing of DHS paid for by Medicare or any other payor (and such non-DHS services must constitute the full array of non-DHS services the physician "routinely" provides).[132]

- The DHS is billed by the group or its billing agent under the group's billing number (though, in certain circumstances, alternative billing arrangements are permitted).[133]

- The DHS does not include DME precluded from protection under this exception or parenteral or enteral nutrients, equipment, or supplies.[134]

Investor Referrals to Fellow Joint Venture Investors. A physician's investment in a joint venture will not, in and of itself, give rise to a financial relationship between him or her and any hospital, physician, or other health care

Investor Referrals to Fellow Joint Venture Investors

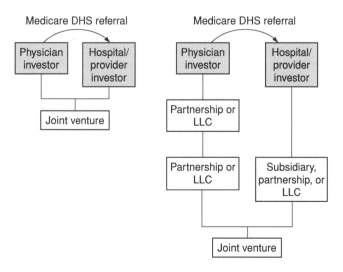

provider or supplier investing in the joint venture. (See accompanying diagram.)[135] Thus, mere co-ownership of a joint venture by a physician and a DHS entity will not—in isolation—preclude Medicare referrals from the investing physician to the investing DHS entity.[136]

Investor Referrals to Those Compensating the Joint Venture. In relatively rare circumstances, a physician investor might incur a financial relationship with a health care provider compensating the joint venture ("Compensating Health Care Provider"). (See the accompanying diagram.) This will most likely arise when (1) the joint venture contracts to furnish items, services, or equipment to the Compensating Health Care Provider, (2) the Compensating Health Care Provider uses such items, services, or equipment in furnishing DHS, and (3) the Compensating Health Care Provider pays the joint venture for each incremental item, incremental unit of service, or incremental use of equipment. Under such circumstances, the physician investor will incur a financial relationship with the Compensating Health Care Provider in the form of an "indirect compensation arrangement."[137] Therefore, the physician will be precluded from referring Medicare beneficiaries to the Compensating Health Care Provider for DHS, and the Compensating Health Care Provider will be prohibited from billing for any DHS furnished pursuant to such a referral (assuming it acts with reckless disregard of the fact that the physician investor receives payment that varies with the volume or value of business generated for the Compensating Health Care Provider) unless one of the following exceptions applies:

- **Qualified Indirect Compensation Arrangement:** The arrangement is limited to a qualified indirect compensation arrangement.[138]

- **Personally Furnished Services:** The investing physician "personally furnishes" any DHS provided to the patient by the Compensating Health Care Provider.[139]

Investor Referrals to Those Compensating the Joint Venture

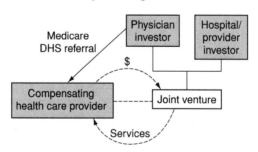

- **Qualified DHS:** The DHS furnished to the Medicare beneficiary by the Compensating Health Care Provider is limited to Qualified DHS.[140]

- **Qualified Prepaid Health Plan Services.** The Medicare beneficiary is enrolled in a qualified "prepaid health plan."[141]

- **Qualified Group Practice Services.** The Compensating Health Care Provider is the referring physician's "group practice,"[142] and the DHS is physician services furnished in accord with the Group Practice Exception.[143]

- **Qualified In-Office Ancillary Services.** The Compensating Health Care Provider is the referring physician's "group practice,"[144] and the DHS is protected by the In-Office Ancillary Services Exception.[145]

Although the law is less clear, DHS referrals might also be permissible if the relationship between the joint venture and Compensating Health Care Provider is limited to a qualified lease of space or equipment,[146] or a qualified personal services arrangement.[147]

Financial Relationships Involving Those Compensated by the Joint Venture

Unless appropriate safeguards are observed, a joint venture might create a financial relationship with those physicians to whom it provides compensation (in cash or kind). The joint venture might preclude (1) the compensated physician from referring Medicare patients to the joint venture for DHS and (2) the joint venture from billing for any DHS provided pursuant to such a referral. This can occur with respect to physicians directly or indirectly compensated by the joint venture.

Referrals to the Joint Venture from Physicians Directly Compensated by the Joint Venture. A physician receiving any payment or benefit (in cash or in kind) from the joint venture ("Compensated Physician") will be deemed to have a "financial relationship" with the joint venture in the form of a "direct compensation arrangement."[148] (See the accompanying diagram.) Consequently, the physician will be precluded from referring Medicare beneficiaries to the joint venture for DHS (and the joint venture will be prohibited from billing for DHS furnished pursuant to such a referral, assuming it acts in reckless disregard of the physician's compensation arrangement) unless one of the following applies:

- **Qualified Compensation Arrangements.** The arrangement between the joint venture and Compensated Physician is limited to a qualified personal services arrangement,[149] a qualified employment arrangement,[150] a qualified physician purchase arrangement,[151] or a qualified fair market value transaction.[152]

Referrals to the Joint Venture from Physicians Directly Compensated by the Joint Venture

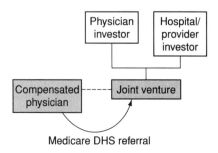

Medicare DHS referral

- **Personally Furnished Services.** The Compensated Physician "personally furnishes" any DHS provided to the patient at the joint venture.[153]

- **Qualified DHS.** The DHS furnished to the Medicare beneficiary is limited to Qualified DHS.[154]

- **Qualified Prepaid Health Plan Services.** The Medicare beneficiary is enrolled in a qualified "prepaid health plan."[155]

- **Qualified Group Practice Services.** The joint venture is a physician "group practice,"[156] and the DHS is physician services furnished in accord with the Group Practice Exception.[157]

- **Qualified In-Office Ancillary Services.** The joint venture is a physician "group practice,"[158] and the DHS is protected by the In-Office Ancillary Services Exception.[159]

Referrals to the Joint Venture from Physicians Indirectly Compensated by the Joint Venture. CMS will deem a physician to have a "financial relationship" with the joint venture in the form of an "indirect compensation arrangement" if (1) there is an unbroken chain of one or more persons between the physician and the joint venture, (2) the compensation received by the physician from the person with whom he or she has a direct relationship varies with the volume or value of referrals or other business the physician generates for the joint venture, and (3) the joint venture has actual

Referrals to the Joint Venture from Physicians Indirectly Compensated by the Joint Venture

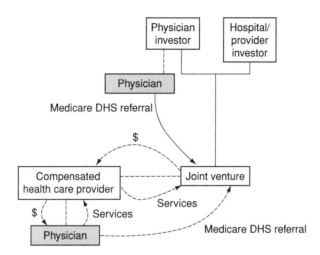

knowledge or acts in reckless disregard or deliberate ignorance of the fact that the physician's compensation varies in such a manner.[160] (See the accompanying diagram.) Consequently, the physician will be precluded from referring Medicare beneficiaries to the joint venture for DHS, and the joint venture will be precluded from billing Medicare for such DHS, unless one of the following applies:

- **Qualified Indirect Compensation Arrangement.** The arrangement between the joint venture and Compensated Physician is limited to a qualified indirect compensation arrangement.[161]

- **Personally Furnished Services.** The Compensated Physician "personally furnishes" any DHS provided to the patient at the joint venture.[162]

- **Qualified DHS.** The DHS furnished to the Medicare beneficiary is limited to Qualified DHS.[163]

- **Qualified Prepaid Health Plan Services.** The Medicare beneficiary is enrolled in a qualified "prepaid health plan."[164]

EXCLUSION LAW

General Provisions

HHS has discretion to exclude any entity from participation in a Federal Program if a person maintaining 5% or greater ownership or control interest in the entity or a person acting as an officer, director, agent, or managing employee of the entity has been (1) convicted of certain enumerated crimes relating to health care billing, patient abuse, substance abuse, or obstruction of a state or federal investigation, (2) held liable for civil money penalties under the Social Security Act, or (3) excluded from participation in a Federal Program.[165] Moreover, if a person "arranges or contracts" with an individual or entity for the provision of items or services that may be paid for by a Federal Program, and such person "knows or should know" that the individual or entity has been excluded from participation in Federal Programs, HHS may (1) impose a $10,000 civil money penalty, (2) impose an assessment of three times the amount of each item or service furnished to a Federal Program beneficiary by the excluded person, and (3) exclude the person contracting with the excluded party from participation in Federal Programs.[166] These sanctions can be imposed even when the excluded person is retained only to provide "administrative and management services" which, though "not directly related to patient care," are "a necessary component" of furnishing covered items or services or are directly or indirectly reimbursed through Federal Program funds.[167]

Application to Joint Ventures

Joint ventures directly or indirectly involved in the furnishing of health care services must abide by the foregoing requirements. This will necessitate the adoption of safeguards to (1) screen potential investors, contractors, and employees for exclusion, (2) screen existing investors, contractors, and employees for exclusion on a periodic basis, and (3) mandate that investors, contractors, and employees immediately inform the joint venture if they are excluded from Federal Programs. Observance of such safeguards should substantially reduce any liability under the Exclusion Law.

ENDNOTES

1. The term "Federal Program," as used throughout this work, refers to Medicare, Medicaid, Tricare, and any other program—with the exception of the Federal Employee Health Benefits Program—that is operated with federal funds. 42 U.S.C. § 1320a–7b(f).

2. Many states have adopted fraud and abuse restrictions which may be implicated by a joint venture arrangement. Although such laws are beyond the scope of this work, special care must be taken to ensure compliance with these state restrictions.

3. 42 U.S.C. § 1320a–7b(b)(2).

4. 42 U.S.C. § 1320a–7b(b)(1).

5. 56 Fed. Reg. 35952, 35958 (1991).

6. *Hanlester Network v. Shalala*, 51 F.3d 1390, 1398 (9th Cir. 1995).

7. *United States v. Kats*, 871 F.2d 105, 108 (9th Cir. 1989).

8. 42 U.S.C. §§ 1320a–7b(b)(1)–(2), 1320a–7(a)(1).

9. 42 U.S.C. §§ 1320a–7a(a)(7), 1320a–7(b)(7).

10. See 42 U.S.C. § 1320a–7b(b)(3) (listing the statutory exceptions to the Anti-Kickback Law); 42 C.F.R. § 1001.952 (listing the regulatory safe harbors to the Anti-Kickback Law).

11. OIG Advisory Opinion 01–17 (Oct. 10, 2001) at 6; 56 Fed. Reg. at 35954.

12. OIG Advisory Opinion 98-4 (April 15, 1998) at 4–5; OIG Advisory Opinion 97–5 (Oct. 6, 1997) at 7. See also 64 Fed. Reg. 63518, 63521 (1999); 56 Fed. Reg. at 35954 (same).

13. 64 Fed. Reg. at 63521 (describing the effect of failure to qualify for safe harbor protection); 56 Fed. Reg. at 35954.

14. 42 U.S.C. § 1320a–7d(a)(2); 66 Fed. Reg. 65460, 65461 (2001); 65 Fed. Reg. 78124, 78125 (2000); 64 Fed. Reg. 69217, 69218-69219 (1999). The foregoing factors are those considered by the OIG in determining whether to issue an advisory opinion protecting an arrangement. One would expect the OIG to utilize the same or similar factors in assessing whether an arrangement under investigation should result in an enforcement action.

15. See 42 U.S.C. § 1320a–7d(b); 42 C.F.R. Part 1008. The requesting parties must pay for all costs incurred by the OIG in issuing the advisory opinion (e.g., personnel, administrative expenses, and so forth).

16. OIG Advisory Opinion 97–5 at 7; 56 Fed. Reg. at 35966–35967.

17. OIG Special Fraud Alert (August 1989), reprinted in 59 Fed. Reg. 65372, 65373 (1994) ("Joint Venture Fraud Alert"); OIG Advisory Opinion 98-12 (Sept. 23, 1998) at 3.

18. OIG Advisory Opinion 01–21 (Nov. 16, 2001) at 6; OIG Advisory Opinion 97-5 at 7. See also 64 Fed. Reg. at 63523 ("We are not persuaded that hospitals, nursing homes, skilled nursing facilities, or other institutions are incapable of influencing referrals of Federal health care program business. To the contrary, we are aware of instances of referrals that are in fact controlled by these institutions' employees or agents."); Financial Arrangements Between Hospitals and Hospital-Based Physicians, OIG Office of Evaluation and Inspection Report No. 9-89-00330 (1989) at 1–2 (concluding that hospitals "can materially influence the flow of Medicare and Medicaid business" and therefore implicate the Anti-Kickback Law).

19. 42 C.F.R. § 1001.952(a)(2). The OIG has also promulgated safe harbors protecting investment interests in large publicly traded entities as well as entities that receive 75% of their annual revenue from patients residing in federally designated underserved areas. See 42 C.F.R. §§ 1001.952(a)(1) (investment safe harbor for certain publicly traded entities), 1001.952(a)(3) (investment safe harbor for entities serving patients located in federally designated medically underserved areas).

20. Joint Venture Fraud Alert at 65374; 56 Fed. Reg. at 35967-359671.

21. 42 C.F.R. § 1001.952(a)(2)(i). The joint venture may use any reasonable accounting method to assess compliance with this standard so long as the method is used consistently. 56 Fed. Reg. at 35969. For purposes of this requirement, "equivalent classes" of equity investments may be combined, and equivalent classes of debt instruments may be combined. 64 Fed. Reg. at 63523. Classes of investment interests will be deemed to be "equivalent" so as to permit aggregation only when they "have similar rights with respect to the entity's income and assets, where investors receive equivalent returns in proportion to the amounts invested, and, most importantly, where there is no preferential treatment of referral source investors, including, but not limited to, preferences that take effect in the event of a disposition of the entity's assets." 64 Fed. Reg. at 63523. The fact that one class of securities is held by passive investors and another class of securities is held by active investors does not preclude qualification as "equivalent" classes so long as the foregoing requirements are met. 59 Fed. Reg. 37202, 37204 (1994). A class of equity investments, however, can never be deemed equivalent with a class of debt investments. 59 Fed. Reg. at 37204.

22. 56 Fed. Reg. at 35969.

23. 42 C.F.R. § 1001.952(a)(4). 56 Fed. Reg. at 35964, 35967, 35969.

24. 42 C.F.R. § 1001.952(a)(2)(ii).

25. 56 Fed. Reg. at 35968.

26. 42 C.F.R. § 1001.952(a)(2)(iii).

27. 56 Fed. Reg. at 35968.

28. 42 C.F.R. § 1001.952(a)(2)(iv).

29. 56 Fed. Reg. at 35969.

30. 42 C.F.R. § 1001.952(a)(2)(v) (parentheses in original). In light of this restriction, the OIG contends that a joint venture seeking protection under the provisions of Investment Interests Safe Harbor may not (1) "use a separate marketing approach or provide a different level of service to passive investors as opposed to noninvestors," (2) appeal to an investor's status as an investor when marketing the joint venture, and (3) "offer special arrangements to investors that are not available or are offered on different terms to noninvestors." 56 Fed. Reg. at 35966.

31. 42 C.F.R. § 1001.952(a)(2)(vi). The joint venture may use any reasonable accounting method to assess compliance with this standard so long as the method is used consistently. 56 Fed. Reg. at 35969.

32. 56 Fed. Reg. at 35969.

33. 42 C.F.R. § 1001.952(a)(4); 56 Fed. Reg. at 35964, 35967, 35969.

34. 42 C.F.R. § 1001.952(a)(2)(vii). This provision does not preclude the joint venture from borrowing funds from one or more investors to cover capital or operating expenses. 56 Fed. Reg. at 35970.

35. 56 Fed. Reg. at 35970.

36. 42 C.F.R. § 1001.952(a)(2)(viii).

37. 42 C.F.R. § 1001.952(a)(4); 56 Fed. Reg. at 35964, 35967, 35969.

38. 42 C.F.R. § 1001.952(a)(4).

39. 42 C.F.R. § 1001.952(a)(4).

40. 42 C.F.R. § 1001.952(r)(4). See 64 Fed. Reg. at 63536, 63538 (providing that distributions from ASC joint ventures that do not meet the ASC Safe Harbor provisions may still qualify for protection under the Investment Interests Safe Harbor). The OIG has also promulgated separate safe harbors for "Surgeon-Owned ASCs," "Single-Specialty ASCs," and "Multi-Specialty ASCs." See 42 C.F.R. § 1001.952(r)(1)–(3). Given the scope of this work, we focus exclusively on the safe harbor governing "Hospital-Physician ASCs."

41. 64 Fed. Reg. at 63536.

42. 64 Fed. Reg. at 63536. See also OIG Advisory Opinion 03-5 (Feb. 6, 2003) (describing concerns with cross-referral arrangements).

43. 58 Fed. Reg. 49008, 49009 (1993); 64 Fed. Reg. at 63534.

44. 64 Fed. Reg. at 63536. "In contrast to other investment interest safe harbors which seek to limit investment by individuals in a position to refer, this proposed ASC safe harbor only protects entities whose investment interests are held *entirely* by such individuals." 58 Fed. Reg. at 49009; 64 Fed. Reg. at 63534 (emphasis in original).

45. 64 Fed. Reg. at 63537-63538. See also OIG Advisory Opinion 98-12 at 4 (describing the government's recognition of the cost-effectiveness of ASCs). The OIG explicitly states that investment by physicians or physicians and hospitals in "non-ASC clinical joint ventures . . . do not share the same policy background and are not subject to the same reimbursement structure as investments by physicians in ASCs." 64 Fed. Reg. at 63538.

46. 42 C.F.R. § 1001.952(r); 64 Fed. Reg. at 63538.

47. 42 C.F.R. § 1001.952(r).

48. 64 Fed. Reg. at 63535, 63538.

49. 42 C.F.R. § 1001.952(r).

50. 64 Fed. Reg. at 63536.

51. 42 C.F.R. § 1001.952(r)(4)(i).

52. 42 C.F.R. § 1001.952(r)(4)(ii).

53. 42 C.F.R. § 1001.952(r)(4)(iii).

54. 42 C.F.R. § 1001.952(r)(4)(iv). This provision does not prevent a physician from refusing to accept new patients, so long as such refusal applies to all private-pay, self-pay, and Federal Program beneficiaries. 64 Fed. Reg. at 63538. Moreover, an ASC is not required to make an affirmative showing that its payer case mix precisely reflects that prevailing in its service area. 64 Fed. Reg. at 63538.

55. 42 C.F.R. § 1001.952(r)(4)(v); 64 Fed. Reg. at 63538.

56. 42 C.F.R. § 1001.952(r)(4)(v); 64 Fed. Reg. at 63538.

57. 42 C.F.R. § 1001.952(r)(4)(v); 64 Fed. Reg. at 63538.

58. 42 C.F.R. § 1001.952(r)(4)(vi). Thus, the safe harbor will not protect distributions from "ancillary services joint ventures married to ASCs." 64 Fed. Reg. at 63539.

59. 42 C.F.R. § 1001.952(r)(4)(vii). The hospital investor is generally precluded from including any costs associated with "developing or operating the ASC" on any Federal Program cost report. 64 Fed. Reg. at 63538. This safeguard is designed to ensure that the hospital does not obtain indirect reimbursement through its cost report for expenses incurred in connection with the ASC joint venture. 64 Fed. Reg. at 63538.

60. 42 C.F.R. § 1001.952(r)(4)(viii).

61. 64 Fed. Reg. at 63537.

62. See OIG Advisory Opinion 03–2 (Jan. 13, 2003) at 8; OIG Advisory Opinion 01-21 at 10; OIG Advisory Opinion 01-17 at 7; OIG Advisory Opinion 97–5 at 7.

63. A person who would typically be deemed to be in a position to refer patients or furnish items or services to the joint venture ASC or joint venture investors may secure exclusion from such status by (1) executing a written stipulation that he or she will not do so and (2) abiding by such stipulation for the life of his or her investment. 64 Fed. Reg. at 63537.

64. 42 C.F.R. § 1001.952(r)(4) (cross referencing 42 C.F.R. § 1001.952(r)(1)).

65. 42 C.F.R. § 1001.952(r)(4) (cross referencing 42 C.F.R. § 1001.952(r)(2)).

66. 42 C.F.R. § 1001.952(r)(4) (cross referencing 42 C.F.R. § 1001.952(r)(3)). The additional requirement that a physician perform at least one-third of his or her ASC-Approved procedures at the joint venture ASC is designed to (1) ensure that the facility serves as an extension of the physician's office and (2) minimize the risk of cross-referral arrangements between physicians in separate specialties. 64 Fed. Reg. at 63537. For example, the requirement would prevent safe harbor protection if an orthopedic surgical group and a pain management anesthesia group exchanged interests in each other's respective ASC joint ventures in order to induce referrals across medical specialties.

67. 42 C.F.R. § 1001.952(r)(5). See also 64 Fed. Reg. at 63536.

68. 42 C.F.R. § 1001.952(r)(5).

69. 64 Fed. Reg. at 63537.

70. OIG Advisory Opinion 97-5 at 5; 56 Fed. Reg. at 35967.

71. See Chapters 7 and 9 of this handbook.

72. 54 Fed. Reg. 3088, 3090-3091 (1989).

73. 42 C.F.R. §§ 1001.952(b)(1), 1001.952(c)(1).

74. 42 C.F.R. §§ 1001.952(b)(2), 1001.952(c)(2).

75. 42 C.F.R. §§ 1001.952(b)(3), 1001.952(c)(3).

76. 64 Fed. Reg. at 63526.

77. 42 C.F.R. §§ 1001.952(b)(4), 1001.952(c)(4).

78. 56 Fed. Reg. at 35973.

79. 64 Fed. Reg. at 63526; OIG Advisory Opinion 01-21 at 10.

80. 42 C.F.R. §§ 1001.952(b)(5), 1001.952(c)(5).

81. 56 Fed. Reg. at 35973.

82. 42 C.F.R. §§ 1001.952(b)(6), 1001.952(c)(6). The term "commercially reasonable business purpose" means "a purpose reasonably calculated to further the business of the lessee or purchaser" (i.e., "the rental or the purchase must be of space, equipment, or services that the lessee or purchaser needs, intends to utilize, and does utilize in furtherance of its commercially reasonable business objectives."). 64 Fed. Reg. at 63525.

83. 64 Fed. Reg. at 63525.

84. 42 C.F.R. § 1001.952(b).

85. 42 C.F.R. § 1001.952(c).

86. 42 C.F.R. § 1001.952(i). For purposes of the Employee Safe Harbor, the term "employee" has the same meaning as it does under the Internal Revenue Code. 42 C.F.R. § 1001.952(i) (cross referencing 26 U.S.C. 3121(d)(2)).

87. 42 C.F.R. § 1001.952(d)(1).

88. 42 C.F.R. § 1001.952(d)(2). For purposes of the Personal Services Safe Harbor, an "agent" of a "principal" is any person, other than a bona fide employee of the principal, who has an agreement to perform services for, or on behalf of, the principal. 42 C.F.R. § 1001.952(d).

89. 42 C.F.R. § 1001.952(d)(3).

90. 64 Fed. Reg. at 63526.

91. 42 C.F.R. § 1001.952(d)(4).

92. 56 Fed. Reg. at 35973.

93. 64 Fed. Reg. at 63526; OIG Advisory Opinion 01-21 at 10.

94. 42 C.F.R. § 1001.952(d)(5).

95. 56 Fed. Reg. at 35973.

96. 56 Fed. Reg. at 35973.

97. 42 C.F.R. § 1001.952(d)(7).

98. 64 Fed. Reg. at 63525. The term "commercially reasonable business purpose" means "a purpose reasonably calculated to further the business of the lessee or purchaser" (i.e., "the rental or the purchase must be of space, equipment, or services that the lessee or purchaser needs, intends to utilize, and does utilize in furtherance of its commercially reasonable business objectives."). 64 Fed. Reg. at 63525.

99. 42 C.F.R. § 1001.952(d)(6).

100. OIG Advisory Opinion 97-5 at 5; 56 Fed. Reg. at 35967.

101. 54 Fed. Reg. at 3090-3091.

102. 63 Fed. Reg. 1659, 1662 (1998).

103. 42 U.S.C. § 1395nn(a)(1)(A); 42 C.F.R. § 411.353(a). CMS has also announced its intention to issue regulations implementing § 1903 of the Social Security Act by denying federal financial participation to state Medicaid programs for DHS furnished pursuant to a referral that would have been prohibited under the Stark Law had the patient been a Medicare beneficiary. 66 Fed. Reg. 856, 859 (2001).

104. 42 U.S.C. § 1395nn(h)(6); 42 C.F.R. § 411.351 (defining the term "designated health services").

105. 42 U.S.C. § 1395nn(h)(5); 42 C.F.R. § 411.351 (defining the term "referral").

106. 42 U.S.C. § 1395nn(h)(5)(C); 42 C.F.R. § 411.351 (defining the term "referral").

107. 42 U.S.C. § 1395nn(h)(5)(C); 42 C.F.R. § 411.351 (defining the term "referral").

108. 42 U.S.C. § 1395nn(h)(5)(C); 42 C.F.R. § 411.351 (defining the term "referral").

109. 42 U.S.C. § 1395nn(a)(1)(B); 42 C.F.R. § 411.353(b).

110. 42 U.S.C. § 1395nn(g)(2).

111. 42 U.S.C. § 1395nn(g)(3).

112. 42 U.S.C. § 1395nn(g)(4). In addition, a physician or entity participating in a "scheme" to circumvent the Stark Law is subject to a civil money penalty of up to $100,000 and exclusion from participation in Federal Programs. 42 U.S.C. § 1395nn(g)(4).

113. See Chapters 8 and 9 in this handbook.

114. 42 U.S.C. § 1395nn(a)(2); 42 C.F.R. § 411.354(b).

115. 42 C.F.R. § 411.354(b).

116. As noted above, the Stark Law provides that, under such circumstances, no referral has occurred so as to implicate the law. See note 105.

117. 42 C.F.R. § 411.355(d).

118. 42 C.F.R. § 411.355(g). The list of drugs covered by this exception is updated annually and published on the CMS web site. 42 C.F.R. § 411.355(g). The arrangement for administration or dispensation of the drug must not violate the Anti-Kickback Law. 42 C.F.R. § 411.355(g)(2). Moreover, billing and claim submission for the drugs must be completed in accord with federal and state law. 42 C.F.R. § 411.355(g)(3).

119. 42 C.F.R. § 411.355(h). The list of preventive tests, immunizations, and vaccines covered by this exception is updated annually and published on the CMS web site. 42 C.F.R. § 411.355(h)(5). The arrangement for provision of these items must not violate the Anti-Kickback Law. 42 C.F.R. § 411.355(h)(3). Moreover, billing and claim submission must be completed in accord with federal and state law. 42 C.F.R. § 411.355(h)(4).

120. 42 C.F.R. § 411.355(i). The arrangement for the furnishing of the eyeglasses and contact lenses must not violate the Anti-Kickback Law. 42 C.F.R. § 411.355(i)(2). Moreover, billing and claim submission must be completed in accord with federal and state law. 42 C.F.R. § 411.355(i)(3).

121. 42 C.F.R. § 411.355(f). The arrangement for provision of the implants must not violate the Anti-Kickback Law. 42 C.F.R. § 411.355(f)(3). Moreover, billing and claim submission must be completed in accord with federal and state law. 42 C.F.R. § 411.355(f)(4).

122. 42 U.S.C. § 1395nn(b)(3); 42 C.F.R. § 411.355(c).

123. 42 U.S.C. § 1395nn(b)(3); 42 C.F.R. § 411.355(c).

124. 42 U.S.C. § 1395nn(d)(3); 42 C.F.R. § 411.356(c)(3). If the hospital is located in Puerto Rico, more liberal restrictions apply. Specifically, the Investing Physician need not have privileges there, and his or her investment interest may be in a subdivision or department of the facility. 42 U.S.C. § 1395nn(d)(1); 42 C.F.R. § 411.356(c)(2).

125. 42 U.S.C. § 1395nn(d)(2). For purposes of this exception, the term "rural" means an area designated as rural for purposes of calculating the standardized amount for hospitals located in the area under the Medicare inpatient prospective payment system for acute care hospitals. 42 U.S.C. § 1395nn(d)(2).

126. 42 U.S.C. §§ 1395nn(b)(1), 1395nn(h)(4), 1395nn (h)(5)(A); 42 C.F.R. §§ 411.352, 411.355(a). An independent contractor must furnish the service during the time in which he or she is under contract to perform patient care services to the Group's patients in the Group's facilities. See 42 C.F.R. §§ 411.355(b)(1)(iii) (permitting Medicare services to be furnished by a "physician in the group practice"), 411.351 (defining "physician in the group practice"). Thus, an independent contractor physician performing the professional component of MRI services off-site does not qualify for protection under this exception.

127. 42 U.S.C. § 1395nn(h)(4); 42 C.F.R. § 411.352.

128. 66 Fed. Reg. at 899.

129. See previous notes 130–131.

130. 42 C.F.R. § 411.355(b)(2)(i)(C).

131. 42 U.S.C. § 1395nn(b)(2)(A)(i); 42 C.F.R. § 411.355(b)(1). A physician contractor must discharge supervision during the time he or she is furnishing patient care services under a contractual obligation to provide such services to the Group's patients in the Group's offices. See 42 C.F.R. §§ 411.355(b)(1)(iii) (permitting Medicare supervision to be discharged by a "physician in the group practice"), 411.351 (defining "physician in the group practice").

132. 42 U.S.C. § 1395nn(b)(2)(A)(ii); 42 C.F.R. § 411.355(b)(2)(i)(A)-(B).

133. 42 U.S.C. § 1395nn(b)(2)(B); 42 C.F.R. § 411.355(b)(3).

134. 42 C.F.R. § 411.355(b).

135. 42 C.F.R. § 411.354(b)(2); 66 Fed. Reg. at 870.

136. 42 C.F.R. § 411.354(b)(2). If a hospital, physician, or other health care provider maintains a financial relationship with the joint venture in the form of a compensation arrangement, that arrangement must be separately analyzed in order to determine whether it generates a financial relationship implicating the Stark Law.

137. 42 C.F.R. § 411.354(c)(2). See also 66 Fed. Reg. at 866 (describing how an indirect compensation arises under circumstances akin to those described above). By contrast, when a health care provider furnishes items or services to the joint venture in return for payment, no indirect compensation arrangement will likely arise because the remuneration received by the joint venture in the form of services will not likely vary with or reflect the volume or value of referrals that the investing physician makes to the provider. 42 C.F.R. § 411.354(b)(2)(ii).

138. 42 C.F.R. § 411.357(p). A qualified indirect compensation arrangement arises when compensation paid to the referring physician (1) is fair market value for items or services actually provided, (2) is set in advance (whether as a flat fee or on a per-unit-of-service basis), (3) does not "take into account" the volume or value of referrals or other business generated by the referring physician for the entity furnishing DHS, and (4) does not violate the Anti-Kickback Law or any laws or regulations governing billing or claims submission. Unless the arrangement pursuant to which the physician receives compensation is a bona fide employment relationship, it must be memorialized in a writing signed by the parties, which specifies the terms of the arrangement. 42 C.F.R. § 411.357(p)(2). Where, as here, the physician's indirect compensation

arrangement with the entity furnishing DHS arises solely due to an investment interest in an entity contracting with the DHS entity, CMS will apply the foregoing requirements to the compensation arrangement most proximate to the physician. 66 Fed. Reg. at 867.

139. See note 116.

140. See notes 117–121.

141. See notes 122–123.

142. See notes 126–128.

143. See notes 126–128.

144. See notes 129–134.

145. See notes 129–134.

146. 42 C.F.R. § 411.357(a)-(b). A qualified lease is one that meets each of the following requirements: (1) it is memorialized in a lease agreement signed by the parties, which runs for a term of at least one year, (2) it provides for exclusive use of the space or equipment during the period in which the lessee uses such space or equipment (though a lessee may be charged a pro-rata share for use of common areas in the building in which it leases space), (3) the space or equipment leased does not exceed that "reasonable and necessary" for the lessee's "legitimate business purposes," (4) the lease would be commercially reasonable in an arm's-length transaction between parties who make no referrals, (5) the rental charge is "set in advance" (whether in aggregate or on a per-use basis) at fair market value and does not vary during the agreement based on the volume or value of business between the parties. 42 C.F.R. §§ 411.357(a)-(b), 411.354(d).

147. 42 C.F.R. § 411.357(d). A qualified personal services arrangement is one that meets each of the following requirements: (1) it is memorialized in an agreement signed by the parties, which runs for a term of at least one year, (2) it covers all services to be furnished between the parties, (3) the aggregate services do not exceed those "reasonable and necessary" for the principal's "legitimate business purposes," (4) the agreement would be commercially reasonable in an arm's-length transaction between parties who make no referrals, and (5) the compensation paid in connection with the agreement is "set in advance" (whether in aggregate or on a per-use basis) at fair market value and does not vary during the agreement based on the volume or value of business between the parties. 42 C.F.R. §§ 411.357(d), 411.354(d).

148. See 42 C.F.R. §§ 411.354(c) (defining "compensation arrangement" to mean the furnishing of "remuneration"), 411.351 (defining "remuneration" to include "any payment or other benefit made directly or indirectly, overtly or covertly, in cash or in kind"). It should be noted, however, that the following benefits will not, in isolation, give rise to a compensation arrangement or other financial relationship when conferred upon a physician: (1) forgiveness of amounts owed for inaccurate or mistakenly performed tests or procedures, (2) the correction of minor billing errors, (3) the furnishing of certain nonsurgical devices or supplies used to collect, transport, process, or store specimens, (4) certain items, devices, or supplies used solely to order tests or communicate test results, and (5) certain payments by health plans for physician services furnished to plan beneficiaries. 42 C.F.R. § 411.351 (defining "remuneration").

149. See note 147.

150. 42 C.F.R. § 411.357(c). A qualified employment arrangement is one which meets each of the following requirements: (1) it covers identifiable services to be performed by the

physician, (2) the agreement would be commercially reasonable in an arm's-length transaction between parties who make no referrals, and (3) the compensation paid in connection with the agreement is "set in advance" (whether in aggregate or on a per-use basis) at fair market value and does not vary during the agreement to account for the volume or value of business between the parties. 42 C.F.R. §§ 411.357(c), 411.354(d).

151. 42 C.F.R. § 411.357(i). A qualified physician purchase arrangement is one in which a physician pays fair market value for items or services actually furnished. 42 C.F.R. § 411.357(i). See 42 C.F.R. § 411.351 (defining the term "fair market value").

152. 42 C.F.R. § 411.357(l). A qualified fair market value transaction is one that meets each of the following requirements: (1) it provides for the sale of items or services from a physician or his or her qualified group practice, (2) it is memorialized in an agreement signed by the parties which runs for a fixed term and specifies all services furnished and compensation paid in connection with the arrangement, (3) it is "commercially reasonable" in scope and duration so as to further the "legitimate business purposes" of the parties, (4) it does not violate the Anti-Kickback Law or involve the counseling or promotion of a business arrangement or activity that violates Federal law, (5) the compensation paid in connection with the agreement is "set in advance" (whether in aggregate or on a per-use basis) at fair market value and does not vary during the agreement to account for the volume or value of business between the parties. 42 C.F.R. §§ 411.357(l), 411.354(d). If the arrangement is for a term of less than one year, it can be renewed any number of times within a year of execution of the first arrangement so long as the terms of the arrangement (including, without limitation, the compensation terms) do not change. 42 C.F.R. § 411.357(l)(2).

153. See note 116.

154. See notes 117–121.

155. See notes 122–123.

156. See notes 126–128.

157. See notes 126–128.

158. See notes 129–134.

159. See notes 129–134.

160. 42 C.F.R. § 411.354(c)(2).

161. See note 138.

162. See note 116.

163. See notes 117–121.

164. See notes 122–123.

165. 42 U.S.C. § 1320a-7(b)(8).

166. 42 U.S.C. § 1320a-7a(a)(6).

167. See OIG Special Advisory Bulletin, "The Effect of Exclusion From Participation In Federal Health Care Programs" (Sept. 1999) (reprinted at 64 Fed. Reg. 58851 (1999)); OIG Advisory Opinion 01-16 (Sept. 28, 2001).

CHAPTER 3

Federal Tax Laws Governing Hospital Joint Ventures

INTRODUCTION

Like their proprietary counterparts, nonprofit tax-exempt hospitals have come to rely increasingly on joint ventures as a means to acquire financing, promote physician loyalty, and secure clinical and managerial expertise. Unlike their proprietary counterparts, however, exempt hospitals must ensure that their joint venture arrangements comport with numerous restrictions imposed by the Internal Revenue Service (the "Service"). Violation of these restrictions can lead to loss of exempt status for the hospital, disqualification of the hospital's tax-exempt bonds, corporate tax liability, and excise tax penalties. This chapter describes how exempt hospitals can participate in joint ventures while avoiding the foregoing sanctions. This chapter assumes that the hospital's exempt status is predicated upon designation as a 501(c)(3) "charitable" organization. Therefore, the terms "exempt purpose" and "charitable purpose" are used interchangeably.

PRESERVATION OF EXEMPT STATUS

General Provisions

The vast majority of nonprofit hospitals are 501(c)(3) "charitable" organizations whose charitable purpose, defined by the "community benefit standard," is the "promotion of health" for a broad portion of the community.[1] These institutions are required to observe three general requirements in order to secure and retain their exempt status.

First, the hospital must be "organized" exclusively in furtherance of a charitable purpose.[2] A hospital satisfies this requirement only if its articles of organization limit it to one or more exempt purposes and do not expressly authorize activities not in furtherance of an exempt purpose.[3] For purposes of this requirement, the term "articles of organization" includes the hospital's corporate charter or any other written instrument by which it is created.[4]

Second, the hospital must be "operated" exclusively in furtherance of its charitable purpose.[5] A hospital satisfies this requirement only if it engages "primarily" in charitable activities.[6] Alternatively stated, the hospital must demonstrate that no more than an "insubstantial part of its activities" are in furtherance of a noncharitable purpose.[7]

Third, the hospital must not convey private inurement or impermissible private benefit.[8] The Service takes the position that any private benefit furnished by the exempt hospital must be "qualitatively incidental" (i.e., be a "necessary concomitant of the activity that benefits the public at large") and "quantitatively incidental" (i.e., be "insubstantial when viewed in relationship to the public benefit "conferred by the hospital").[9] Moreover, pursuant to the private inurement restriction, remuneration may be furnished by the exempt hospital to one of the exempt hospital's "insiders" only as part of a commercially reasonable exchange (in other words, an exchange involving terms and payments equivalent to transactions negotiated at arm's length).[10] One commentator has defined the term "insider" to include any person who "has the ability to control or otherwise influence the actions of the tax-exempt organization so as to cause the benefit."[11] Notably, the Service has conceded that a physician does not become an "insider" at an exempt hospital merely by securing staff privileges at the facility.[12]

Application to a Hospital Joint Venture

The question arises as to whether and under what circumstances a hospital jeopardizes its exempt status by participation in a joint venture, particularly when one or more of the venturers are not § 501(c)(3) organizations. Specifically, the question becomes: Does such activity (1) indicate that the hospital is no longer operated "exclusively for charitable purposes" or (2) result in the transfer of private inurement or impermissible private benefit to fellow joint venture participants or third parties? The analysis varies substantially depending upon how the joint venture is structured.

Use of a Flow-Through Entity

When it can do so without jeopardizing its exempt status, a hospital will most often choose to organize a joint venture as a partnership, limited partnership, or limited liability company treated as a partnership for tax purposes (collectively referred to as "Flow-Through Entities").[13] Flow-Through Entities are a preferable vehicle for joint venture arrangements because they pay no tax themselves; rather, they serve as a conduit through which income, losses, and other tax benefits are allotted to investors for taxation at their respective tax rates. Since an exempt hospital generally pays no income tax, it can often retain the entire "pretax" value of the distributions it receives from the joint venture.[14] For-profit partners benefit from such a structure because they avoid double taxation on joint venture proceeds.

The operative question, then, is precisely when and under what circumstances can an exempt hospital participate in a joint venture structured as a Flow-Through Entity without jeopardizing its exempt status. An exempt hospital may serve as a passive investor (i.e., a limited partner or nonmanaging LLC member) in a joint venture structured as a Flow-Through Entity without jeopardizing its exempt status so long as (1) the investment is prudent and (2) the exempt hospital's share of distributed or undistributed revenue from activity "unrelated" to its charitable purpose is not too substantial when compared to its overall charitable activities.[15] When the exempt hospital serves as an active investor (in other words, as a general partner or managing LLC member), however, the analysis differs. Under such circumstances, the business activity of the joint venture is imputed directly to the hospital.[16] Therefore, the joint venture will jeopardize the hospital's exemption unless federal courts and the Service determine that the joint venture (1) furthers the hospital's exempt purpose, (2) allows the hospital to operate exclusively for exempt purposes, and (3) is devoid of private inurement or excess private benefit.[17] Each such requirement is addressed in the sections that follow.

The Joint Venture Must Further the Hospital's Charitable Purpose. The Service will first inquire whether participation in the joint venture furthers the hospital's exempt purpose.[18] As noted above, the vast majority of nonprofit hospitals are 501(c)(3) "charitable" organizations whose exempt purpose, defined by the "community benefit" standard, is the "promotion of health" for a broad portion of the community.[19] The Service has traditionally been most amenable to finding community benefit (and, therefore, exempt purpose) in joint ventures formed for (1) "creation of a new provider of health care services," (2) "expansion of community health care services," (3) "improvement in treatment modalities," (4) "reduction in health care costs," and (5) "improved patient convenience and access to physicians."[20] The Service has explicitly concluded that joint ventures further a charitable purpose when created to establish or maintain the following facilities for use by a broad section of the community:

- A rehabilitation hospital.[21]

- A psychiatric hospital.[22]

- An acute care hospital.[23]

- A nursing home.[24]

- An outpatient physical therapy clinic.[25]

- An ambulatory surgery center.[26]

- A diagnostic imaging facility.[27]

- A women's health clinic.[28]

- A lithotripsy facility.[29]

- An outpatient dialysis center.[30]

- An outpatient cardiac diagnostic services clinic.[31]

- A home health care agency.[32]

- A medical office building adjacent to the hospital campus in which space is made available to physicians on the hospital staff. [33]

- An eldercare facility.[34]

- A cancer treatment center or radiation oncology facility.[35]

- A medical clinic located in an underserved area and treating all patients regardless of ability to pay.[36]

Any such facility must be made available to Medicare and Medicaid beneficiaries.[37]

The Service has also concluded that, although certain components of integrated delivery systems such as physician–hospital organizations ("PHOs") and management services organizations ("MSOs") cannot independently qualify as exempt entities under the community benefit standard, an exempt hospital will not likely jeopardize its charitable status by participating in a PHO or MSO joint venture structured as a Flow-Through Entity so long as the hospital maintains adequate control over the joint venture and prevents private inurement or impermissible private benefit.[38] An exempt hospital will best protect itself by documenting the general cost-savings and clinical benefits associated with the integration arrangement.[39]

The Joint Venture Must Not Impede the Hospital's Ability to Operate Exclusively for Exempt Purposes. Upon establishing that a joint venture generally furthers the exempt hospital's charitable purpose, the Service will inquire whether the joint venture might nonetheless interfere with the hospital's ability to operate exclusively in furtherance of that purpose.[40] Specifically, once it participates in the joint venture, can the hospital still be said to (1) engage "primarily" in activities which meet the community benefit standard or other exempt purpose and (2) ensure that only an insubstantial portion (if any) of its activities are in furtherance of a nonexempt purpose?[41] In making this assessment, federal courts and the Service focus on the "purpose" rather than the "nature" of the hospital's activities. Thus, the mere fact that a hospital engages in a trade or business through a joint venture will not jeopardize its exempt status so long as these activities are undertaken to further its charitable purpose.[42] Nonetheless, if the hospital maintains even a single substantial nonexempt purpose in undertaking the joint venture, it will jeopardize its exemption regardless of the number or importance of exempt purposes.[43] The Service has historically expressed three principal concerns when analyzing whether a hospital's participation in a joint venture will preclude it from operating exclusively for exempt purposes. These three—protection of exempt assets, reconciliation of fiduciary duties, and operational control—are each discussed in the next sections.

Protection of Exempt Assets

The Service will initially scrutinize whether the exempt hospital adequately limits its exposure to financial loss resulting from joint venture activities. The Service has historically been particularly concerned when an exempt hospital acts as a general partner in a joint venture arrangement, contending that its resulting liability under state law for all partnership obligations might interfere with the entity's charitable mission.[44] Under such circumstances, the Service inquires whether the exempt hospital has taken prudent steps to "insulate itself" from excessive liability. Principal means of protection previously recognized by the Service include maintenance of adequate insurance by the joint venture, indemnity agreements from other joint venture participants, use of nonrecourse debt on the part of the joint venture, and omission of any guarantee to reimburse limited partners for their losses in connection with the joint venture.[45] The nature of the joint venture's activities will dictate the degree of protection warranted. When one is structuring a partnership arrangement to limit an exempt hospital's liability for debts resulting from its participation in the joint venture, care should be taken to ensure that such liability restrictions do not subject the partnership to designation as a corporation under § 7701 of the IRC.[46]

Although concerns with exposure of exempt assets will be less pronounced when the exempt hospital serves as a limited partner or LLC member, the Service will heavily scrutinize any contractual pledge by the hospital to assume or guarantee joint venture debts or losses incurred by other joint venture members.[47] Such an arrangement would raise concerns relating to exposure of exempt assets as well as private benefit and private inurement (discussed below). Nonetheless, such an arrangement might be permissible when the guarantee or indemnity is limited in scope and part of a larger commercially reasonable arm's length transaction.[48]

Reconciliation of Fiduciary Duties

Once the exempt hospital's assets are deemed sufficiently insulated from exposure by the joint venture, both the Service and federal courts will inquire whether the hospital reconciles any fiduciary duties owed to fellow joint venture participants with the hospital's charitable mission. Again, the Service's concern has been most pronounced in instances in which an exempt hospital acts as a general partner in a joint venture arrangement, contending that its resulting fiduciary duty under state law to further the commercial interests of fellow investors might conflict with its charitable mission.[49] The Service recognizes, however, that such a conflict can often be resolved through a legally enforceable agreement among joint venture participants that the exempt hospital's charitable purposes supersede any fiduciary obligation it might otherwise have to maximize the joint venture's profits.[50] To the extent that an exempt hospital incurs such a fiduciary duty under applicable state law when acting as a limited partner or LLC member, the Service would likely require a similar agreement.[51]

Operational Control

Once the joint venture's organizational documents are deemed to provide for the primacy of charitable purposes, the Service will scrutinize whether the exempt hospital is granted sufficient operational control to enforce this requirement. Both the Service and federal courts have indicated that adequate control is most readily secured when the hospital maintains a sufficient majority on the venture's governing board to unilaterally (1) set charges for clinical services, (2) terminate or add clinical services lines, (3) terminate management agreements, and (4) make "fundamental operating decisions."[52] According to the Service, fundamental operating decisions subject to board review should include approval of capital and operating budgets, the timing and amount of distributions, selection of key executives, the acquisition or disposition of health care facilities, execution of contracts exceeding a fixed monetary threshold, changes to service mix, and amendment of the governing documents for the joint venture.[53]

Ensuring adequate operational control on the part of the exempt hospital is more difficult in the absence of its outright majority control over joint venture governance. Throughout the 1980s and early 1990s, the Service approved a number of joint ventures in which charitable purposes were made paramount but the exempt hospital maintained only 50% control (and, in a few cases, less than 50% control).[54] Thereafter, the Service appeared to reverse course, more recently arguing that an exempt hospital's numerical control of a joint venture's governing body is all but necessary to ensure the joint venture is operated to serve charitable purposes.[55] This more stringent position has never been explicitly adopted by federal courts. Indeed, a recent seminal precedent, *Redlands Surgical Services v. Commissioner* establishes that outright majority voting power is not a necessary condition to ensure adequate control on the part of an exempt hospital over a joint venture.[56] Nonetheless, it remains unclear precisely what safeguards must be adopted to ensure sufficient control on the part of the exempt hospital in the absence of majority control on the joint venture board. At present, *Redlands* and *St. David's Health Care System v. United States* provide us with the best guidance as to requirements likely to be imposed by federal courts regardless of whether a joint venture is for clinical services or to form an integrated delivery system.[57]

In *Redlands*, the Ninth Circuit denied exempt status to a nonprofit corporation whose sole function was to serve as co-general partner with a for-profit entity in the operation of a surgical center. With voting control split 50-50 between the two general partners, the Ninth Circuit stated "we look to the binding commitments made between [the nonprofit] and the other parties to ascertain whether other specific powers or rights conferred upon the [nonprofit] might mitigate or compensate for its lack of majority control" and otherwise ensure that the joint venture is operated exclusively for charitable purposes.[58] The court ultimately concluded that no such safeguards existed. Nonetheless, in the course of its analysis, the court suggested (by negative implication) that the following factors might collectively be indicative of formal or informal control:

- Matters on which directors are divided are submitted to binding arbitration before independent arbitrators who are obligated to favor charitable purposes over commercial interests in resolving disputes.

- Where a facility is to be operated under management contract, the contract reserves broad oversight powers to the joint venture, runs for a limited term (perhaps 5 years or less), is renewable only upon consent of the exempt hospital, permits for-cause termination by the exempt hospital, includes a binding contractual requirement that the management company favor charitable purposes over profits, and calculates compensation for the management company in a manner that provides no disincentive to charity care (e.g., by a flat-fee payment or a percentage-of-revenue payment that explicitly includes charity care as revenue).[59]

- Where a medical advisory group is used, the group is composed of physicians with no economic interest in the joint venture.[60]

- The exempt hospital reserves the right to implement a quality assurance program for medical care at any facility operated by the joint venture.[61]

- The facility operated by the joint venture furnishes substantial charity care and maintains a substantial Medicaid utilization level.[62]

The subsequent ruling by the Fifth Circuit in *St. David's Health Care System v. United States*, however, adds further confusion as to what — if any — safeguards can be adopted to ensure adequate control by a nonprofit member of a joint venture in the absence of a voting majority on the joint venture's governing body. In *St. David's*, a nonprofit entity contributed its hospital facility to a joint venture with a for profit entity, and the joint venture was managed by a company affiliated with the for-profit partner. The Service concluded that St. David's lacked requisite control over the joint venture to ensure operation exclusively for charitable purposes, and therefore revoked the System's exempt status. Although, control of the joint venture's governing body was split 50-50 between the parties, the joint venture's governing documents included a number a safeguards to protect St. David's charitable mission. Safeguards included:

- A mandate in the partnership agreement requiring that partnership facilities be operated in accordance with the community benefit standard (including acceptance of Medicare and Medicaid patients, treating patients with emergency conditions without regard to ability to pay, maintaining an open medical staff, providing public health programs of educational benefit to the community, and providing "quality health care at a reasonable cost" to thecommunity).

- St. David's explicit right to terminate unilaterally the management agreement if the management company takes any action with a "material probability of adversely affecting" St. David's exempt status.

- Provision that no measure can pass the partnership board without support from a majority of the board members appointed by St. David's.

- St. David's explicit right to appoint the initial CEO for the partnership, subject to the veto of the for-profit partner.

- The explicit right of either St. David's or the for-profit partner to unilaterally remove the CEO.

- St. David's explicit right to initiate dissolution of the partnership if it receives legal advice from an attorney acceptable to both joint venture partners that continued participation in the partnership will hinder St. David's tax-exempt status.[63]

In light of the foregoing safeguards, the trial court had awarded summary judgment to St. David's, ruling that—as a matter of law—St. David's exercised requisite control over the joint venture. However, the Fifth Circuit reversed the trial court decision, ruling that—notwithstanding all of the safeguards enumerated above—there was a jury question as to whether St. David's had ceded such control over the joint venture to its for-profit partner that St. David's was no longer operated exclusively for charitable purposes. In so ruling, the Fifth Circuit questioned whether the above-referenced safeguards would provide St. David's with sufficient effective control over operation of the joint venture to ensure exclusive operation for charitable purposes absent majority voting control. Specifically the Court made the following findings:

- With control of only 50% of the partnership's governing board, St. David's can only "veto"—rather than "initiate"—action through the joint venture in furtherance of St. David's charitable goals.

- The partnership's hospital would be managed — through a long-term contract—by a for-profit management company affiliated with the for-profit joint venture partner and compensated based upon partnership revenues.[64]

- The management agreement might not permit sufficient oversight by the partnership over the daily operation of the partnership's facilities.

- The principal means available to St. David's to ensure supremacy of charitable interests (i.e., termination of the management agreement, litigation with the management company, termination of the CEO, or dissolution of the partnership) were extraordinary steps which might not be take n in response to daily operational concerns involving charitable interests.

Given the recent rulings in Redlands and St. David's, there is substantial ambiguity as to what safeguards would, in the absence of 51% majority voting control, be deemed sufficient to permit an exempt hospital to ensure that a joint venture in which it participates is operated exclusively in furtherance of the hospital's charitable purposes. Thus, pending further guidance from federal courts or the Service, hospitals participating in such ventures—at least those structured as flow-through entities—might deem it advisable to insist on 51% voting control on the governing board and in connection with all major governance decisions. Management contracts for joint venture facilities should also be of limited duration and provide for reasonable oversight of the daily operations of the joint venture.

Private Inurement or Impermissible Private Benefit. An exempt hospital is prohibited from conveying private inurement or impermissible private benefit. Violation of either prohibition will result in loss or denial of exempt status.[65] The "mere fact" that an exempt hospital enters into a joint venture with private parties who receive a return on their capital investment does not establish that the exempt hospital has impermissibly conferred private benefit."[66] Nonetheless, the Service takes the position that any private benefit furnished by the exempt hospital or the joint venture itself must be "qualitatively incidental" (i.e., be a "necessary concomitant of the activity that benefits the public at large") and "quantitatively incidental" (i.e., be "insubstantial when viewed in relationship to the public benefit conferred by the activity.").[67] Moreover, pursuant to the private inurement restriction, remuneration may be furnished by the exempt hospital or the joint venture itself to one of the hospital's "insiders" only as part of a commercially reasonable exchange (i.e., an exchange involving terms and payments equivalent to transactions negotiated at arm's length).[68] As noted above, one commentator has defined the term "insider" to include any person who "has the ability to control or otherwise influence the actions of the tax-exempt organization so as to cause the benefit."[69] On occasion, the Service has indicated that control over a discrete segment of an exempt organization may result in classification as an "insider." As further noticed above, the Service has conceded that a physician does not become an "insider" at an exempt hospital merely by securing staff privileges at the facility.[70]

In general, the Service and federal courts have closely scrutinized the following factors in determining whether a joint venture gives rise to private inurement or impermissible private benefit.

Factors Helpful to Positive Decisions

- Profits and losses are allocated between the joint venture partners or members according to their respective equity interests which, in turn, are proportionate to their respective capital contributions.[71]

- Any financing, assets, guarantees, or services provided by the exempt hospital to the joint venture are furnished at market rates.[72]

- The compensation and other terms in any management contract involving the joint venture are commercially reasonable (i.e., similar to those in similar agreements negotiated at arm's length).[73]

- The joint venture receives fair market value compensation for all items, services, or payments it provides to investors or third parties.[74]

- The exempt hospital receives dissolution distributions equivalent to its capital account balance and equity stake.[75]

- The exempt hospital receives the right to purchase any equipment or facility owned by the joint venture upon termination.[76]

- Any new facility or integrated delivery system created by the joint venture maintains an open medical staff.[77]

- Debt assumed by the exempt hospital upon entry into a pre-existing joint venture is collateralized, nonrecourse debt.[78]

Factors Harmful to a Positive Decision

- "[T]here is a disproportionate allocation of profits and losses to the nonexempt" joint venture participants.[79]

- The exempt hospital makes loans to the joint venture that are "commercially unreasonable" due to a low interest rate, inadequate security, or other commercially unreasonable terms.[80]

- The exempt hospital provides property or services to the joint venture at less than fair market value or pursuant to terms that are not commercially reasonable.[81]

- The joint venture provides goods or services to nonexempt investors or third parties at less than fair market value.[82]

- Risk asymmetry (i.e., the exempt hospital incurs a disproportionately large portion of the joint venture's downside risk or receives a disproportionately limited portion of the joint venture's upside potential).[83]

- Any new facility or integrated delivery system created by the joint venture will be available only to select members of the exempt hospital's medical staff. [84]

- A facility owned by the joint venture is operated under a management contract for an extended term, renewable thereafter at the sole discretion of the management company.[85]

- The exempt hospital executes a covenant not to compete with the joint venture or other ventures sponsored by the nonexempt joint venture participants.[86]

The Service has identified one category of transactions which, in its opinion, results in *per se* private inurement. Specifically, the sale of a gross or net revenue stream in a hospital department to a joint venture comprised in part of staff physicians will likely constitute private inurement), thereby jeopardizing the hospital's exempt status.[87]

Summary. Collectively, the Service and federal courts have provided guidance as to when a joint venture will be deemed to further a charitable purpose, the requisite safeguards that must be adopted to protect the exempt hospital's assets, the necessary protections to ensure that the exempt hospital's fiduciary duties to joint venture participants do not interfere with its charitable mission, and the circumstances under which joint venture activity might result in inurement or impermissible private benefit. Substantial ambiguity remains, however, in identifying the precise safeguards necessary to ensure that an exempt hospital maintains requisite control over joint venture activities in the absence of majority representation on the venture's governing board. In determining the array of appropriate safeguards to ensure sufficient control by the exempt hospital under such circumstances, one must be particularly cautious in connection with disposition arrangements (i.e., arrangements such as a whole-hospital joint venture in which the exempt hospital has pledged all of its assets to the joint venture). The Service would seemingly be more likely to seek revocation of a hospital's exempt status for lack of control over such a joint venture rather than an ancillary services arrangement in which the exempt hospital retains substantial assets and continues furnishing services in its own right in compliance with the community benefit standard.[88]

Use of a Non-Flow-Through Subsidiary

When there is substantial doubt or ambiguity as to whether a joint venture will further an exempt hospital's charitable purpose or doubt as to whether it can be structured so as to ensure the requisite degree of control on the part of the exempt hospital, the hospital may consider creation of a taxable corporate subsidiary, in the form of a C corporation or a limited liability company taxable as a corporation, to participate in the venture.[89] So long as the subsidiary is incorporated and operated for a legitimate business purpose, is treated as a separate legal entity (i.e., corporate formalities are observed such as separate accounts, separate personnel, distinct facilities, and no majority overlap of officers and directors), and is not used by the exempt hospital as a conduit for indirect private inurement, the subsidiary's activities should pose no risk to the parent's exempt status.[90] Moreover, in many cases, use of such a subsidiary affords greater protection to the exempt hospital than a Flow-Through Entity with respect to financial, civil, and criminal liability for the acts of the joint venture. Furthermore, the subsidiary will have access to capital through the equity market as well as greater operational flexibility than an exempt hospital. Finally, post-tax dividend distributions to the exempt hospital will not give rise to unrelated business income liability, as long as the hospital's ownership interest in the subsidiary is not debt-financed.[91]

Likewise, where the activities involve a substantial portion of the exempt hospital's assets or activities, it may wish to secure a private letter ruling regarding continued exempt status from the Service.

UNRELATED BUSINESS INCOME TAX

General Provisions

Notwithstanding its general exemption from federal income tax liability, a hospital with exempt status under § 501(c)(3) will be taxed at corporate rates on the modified gross income it receives in connection with any "trade or business" that it "regularly carries on" and that is not substantially related to its exempt mission.[92] Moreover, excessive unrelated business income could ultimately jeopardize an organization's exempt status.

Identifying Gross Income from Unrelated Business Activities

In determining whether an activity is a "trade or business," the Service will inquire whether it "is carried on for the production of income" from the sale of goods or performance of services.[93] Although the activity must be carried on with a profit objective, it need not actually result in a profit to satisfy this test.[94] Moreover, the mere fact that a trade or business activity is one component of a broader array of related or integrated activities that may collectively be related to a charitable purpose does not mean that the individual activity loses its designation as a business activity.[95] For example, the sale of supplies by a hospital pharmacy to the general public does not lose its identity as a trade or business merely because the pharmacy also furnishes supplies to hospital inpatients in connection with the hospital's exempt mission.[96]

In determining whether a trade or business is "regularly" carried on, the Service will scrutinize the "frequency" and "continuity" of the activity as well as the "manner" in which it is pursued, and thereafter determine whether the activity is "similar to comparable commercial activities" of nonexempt organizations.[97]

Assuming an activity is (1) a trade or business and (2) regularly carried on, the activity will not result in unrelated business taxable income if the activity is "substantially related" to the hospital's exempt purpose.[98] Specifically, the business or trade activity must have a substantial "causal relationship" to the achievement of charitable purposes (other than through mere production of income).[99] Alternatively stated, the activity must "contribute importantly" to the accomplishment of the exempt organization's charitable purpose.[100] In making this determination, the Service is mindful as to whether the trade or business activities are conducted "on a larger scale than is reasonably necessary" for the performance of an organization's exempt functions.[101] If so, that excess will generate gross income potentially subject to taxation.[102]

Making Appropriate Pre-Tax Deductions from and Modifications to Unrelated Taxable Business Income

Once an exempt hospital's gross unrelated taxable income is identified, certain pre-tax adjustments are made. These adjustments come in the form of deductions and modifications. Again, these deductions and modifications are only relevant if the activity that generates the income is (1) a trade or business, (2) regularly carried on, and (3) not substantially related to the hospital's exempt purposes.

Deductions. Permissible deductions generally consist of the following offsets to unrelated business taxable income: (1) a $1,000 "specific deduction," (2) deductible business expenses "directly connected" with the conduct of the business activity generating the unrelated business income, and (3) charitable contributions equivalent to 10% of unrelated business income if such deduction were not made.[103]

Modifications. Once the foregoing deductions are made, the exempt organization is permitted to exclude a number of additional items when calculating its tax liability. These include the following:

- Dividends, interest, annuities, royalties, and substantially similar passive income from certain other ordinary and routine investments.[104]

- Rent from real property (and any associated *incidental* personal property) so long as the rental charge is either (a) a fixed percentage of gross receipts or sales derived from use of the property or (b) determined in a manner which does not account for income or profits derived from such property.[105]

- Gain or loss from the sale, exchange or other disposition of property other than inventory or items primarily held for sale to customers in the ordinary course of business.[106]

- Gains from the expiration of options to buy or sell investment securities.[107]

- Certain research activities.[108]

The foregoing modifications (the "Modifications"), however, are subject to two exceptions.

First, income in the form of interest, annuities, royalties, and rents derived from organizations 50% or more controlled by the exempt organization shall be factored into the exempt organization's unrelated business taxable income if the income would have been "unrelated" to the organization's exempt purpose if earned directly by the exempt entity.[109] This requirement is enforced even where the income derives from an unrelated activity which is not "regularly carried on" by the exempt organization or controlled entity.[110] It should be emphasized that *this rule does not apply to* dividends received from controlled for-profit corporate entities.

Second, the foregoing modifications are reduced to the extent they derive from "debt-financed property" (i.e., property "held to produce income" and subject to "acquisition debt").[111] Generally, the extent to which such income is subject to tax will be equivalent to the extent to which the property is debt-financed. Specifically, unrelated business taxable income is determined by multiplying that gross income from the property by the quotient obtained when dividing the average acquisition indebtedness for the property in the tax year by the average adjusted basis for the property during that time.[112] Deductions directly related to the property are generally allowable in the same proportion.[113] Capital gains on sale of the property will also be subject to similar recognition.[114]

Several categories of debt-financed property, however, are protected from generating unrelated business income. First, property will not be deemed debt-financed property if at least 85% of its use is substantially related to the owner's exempt purpose.[115] Second, property will not be deemed debt-financed property if the gross income derived from it is treated as unrelated taxable business income.[116] Third, the property will not be deemed debt-financed property if the gross income derived from it is limited to research activity excluded from the definition of unrelated business income.[117] Fourth, real property will not be deemed debt-financed property if it is leased by an exempt hospital to a medical clinic primarily for the purpose of promoting health in the community (i.e., for the provision of patient care to the community).[118] Fifth, property owned by an exempt organization and used by a related exempt organization does not constitute debt-financed property to the extent it is used by the related organization to further its charitable purpose.[119] Sixth, property acquired for prospective exempt use is afforded protection under certain circumstances.[120] Finally, certain debt-encumbered properties acquired by gift, bequest, or devise, will be protected from qualifying as debt-financed property for a period after receipt by the exempt organization.[121]

Application to Hospital Joint Ventures

Flow-Through Entity

As noted above, to the extent it can do so without jeopardizing its exempt status, a hospital and its joint venture partners will most often choose to organize a joint venture as a Flow-Through Entity so as to avoid taxation at the joint venture level. The operative question, then, is under what circumstances will an exempt hospital incur unrelated business income tax liability for participating in a joint venture structured in this manner. The answer is as follows: The exempt hospital will incur tax liability on its share of all modified gross income generated by the Flow-Through Entity joint venture from any "trade or business" in which the joint venture is "regularly engaged" and which is not "substantially related to" the exempt hospital's exempt purpose. The hospital will incur this liability irrespective of whether the unrelated income has been distributed to it by the joint venture.[122] If the amount of unrelated business income attributable to the hospital becomes too great, its exempt status will be jeopardized.

The overwhelming majority of hospital-sponsored joint venture arrangements involve the conduct of a "trade or business" on a "regular basis." Thus, the determination as to whether such trade or business is "substantially related" to the hospital's exempt purpose will dictate whether the income is subject to taxation.[123] In order to be substantially related, the joint venture's business or trade activities must have a substantial "causal relationship" with or "contribute importantly" to the hospital's exempt purposes (e.g., furnishing of care to a broad portion of the community).[124] In making this determination, the Service is mindful as to whether the "size and extent" of the trade or business activities are "larger" than "reasonably necessary" for the performance of the hospital's exempt functions.[125] If so, that excess will generate gross income potentially subject to taxation.[126]

Federal statute explicitly provides that any trade or business carried on by an exempt hospital for the convenience of its members, students, patients, officers, or employees must be considered to be substantially related to the hospital's exempt purposes.[127] The term "patient" is defined to include (1) hospital inpatients, (2) hospital outpatients, (3) individuals referred for specific diagnostic or treatment procedures furnished by hospital-affiliated personnel at a hospital facility, (4) residents of a hospital-affiliated extended care facility, (5) those receiving follow-up or pre-admission radiology or laboratory testing, and (6) individuals receiving medical service in their residence in a hospital-administered home care program.[128] The Service has applied the carve-out to conclude that such activities as operation of an on-site parking, cafeteria, or coffee shop for use by hospital patients, visitors, and staff will not generate unrelated business income.[129]

Absent application of the foregoing statutory exception, the Service will apply a facts-and-circumstances test to assess whether joint venture activity is substantially related to the hospital's exempt mission. In doing so, the Service will view favorably any indication that the activity involves the "laying of hands" on a patient for clinical treatment.[130] The Service has applied this standard in concluding that income from the following activities will not generate unrelated business income:

- Joint venture to establish and operate an ambulatory surgery center.[131]

- Joint venture to establish and operate a diagnostic imaging center.[132]

- Joint venture to establish a radiation therapy center.[133]

- Joint venture to establish and operate a long-term care nursing home.[134]

- Joint venture to establish an eldercare facility.[135]

- Joint venture to establish and operate a freestanding women's health center.[136]

- Joint venture to operate an acute care hospital.[137]

- Joint venture to establish and operate an acute care hospital.[138]

- Joint venture to establish and operate a psychiatric hospital.[139]

- Joint venture to operate a rehabilitation hospital.[140]

- Joint venture to establish and operate a rehabilitation hospital.[141]

- Joint venture to renovate and operate an outpatient rehabilitation clinic.[142]

- Joint venture to establish and operate a cardiac diagnostic services facility.[143]

- Joint venture to establish and operate a home health agency.[144]

- Joint venture to establish and operate an outpatient dialysis facility.[145]

- Joint venture to establish a joint operating company to provide management and oversight of hospitals integrated through a virtual merger.[146]

- Joint venture among several proximate exempt hospitals to furnish clinical laboratory services to their respective inpatients and outpatients (but *not* to nonpatients).[147]

It should be noted that the Service has concluded that revenues from an MSO joint venture will not be deemed "substantially" related to an exempt hospital's charitable mission and will therefore generate unrelated business income tax.[148] Revenues derived from a PHO joint venture's services to physicians in private practice are also deemed not to be "substantially" related to an exempt hospital's charitable mission and will therefore generate unrelated business income tax.[149] Revenues derived from PHO services to the exempt hospital and its patients, however, will not give rise to unrelated business income tax because they are deemed to qualify for the statutory exemption described above.[150]

Once an exempt hospital's gross income from unrelated joint venture business activities is identified, pre-tax deductions and modifications are made. As noted above, permissible deductions generally consist of the following offsets to unrelated business taxable income: (1) a $1,000 "specific deduction," (2) deductible business expenses "directly connected" with the conduct of the business activity generating the unrelated business income, and (3) charitable contributions equivalent to 5% or less unrelated business income if such deduction were not made.[151] The net operating loss deduction provided by IRC § 172 is allowed as an offset to unrelated business taxable income.[152] The net operating loss carryover, however, shall be determined without taking into account the "specific deduction" or any income or deduction that is not included under § 511 in computing unrelated business taxable income.[153] Once these deductions are made, numerous additional modifications must be made.[154]

Non-Flow-Through Entity

If a joint venture will be regularly engaged in a trade or business unrelated to the exempt hospital's charitable purpose, the hospital should give strong consideration to structuring the joint venture as a C corporation or LLC taxed as a corporation. Although the joint venture's activities will be taxed at the subsidiary level, neither income received nor distributions paid by the subsidiary will generate unrelated business income for the hospital.[155] One caveat, however, is worth noting. Interest, annuities, royalties, and rents received by the exempt hospital from the subsidiary and unrelated to the hospital's exempt purpose will generate unrelated business income if the hospital maintains 50% or greater control over the subsidiary, or if the income-generating property is debt-financed.[156] This requirement is enforced even where the income derives from an unrelated activity that is not "regularly carried on" by the exempt hospital or the joint venture subsidiary.[157]

RESTRICTIONS ON THE USE OF TAX-EXEMPT BOND PROCEEDS

General Provisions

Many exempt hospitals rely upon proceeds from "qualified 501(c)(3) bonds" as a source of comparatively low-cost capital for financing capital improvements.[158] The interest paid by the hospital on such bonds is excludable by the recipient for federal (and often state and local) income tax purposes.[159] Consequently, investors accept a lower interest rate than would be demanded on a taxable investment instrument.[160]

Exclusion of interest payments by bondholders is predicated upon the exempt hospital's ongoing compliance with several requirements.[161] First, any property financed with bond proceeds must be owned exclusively by the exempt hospital (or a governmental unit).[162] Second, no more than 5% of the "net proceeds" of a bond issue made after 1986 may be devoted to a nonqualifying use, and payment of the principal or interest on no more than 5% of the net proceeds of an issue may be directly or indirectly related to property put to a nonqualifying use.[163] A "nonqualifying use" includes (1) any direct or indirect use of bond proceeds by a person other than the hospital and (2) the direct or indirect use of bond proceeds by the exempt hospital for an activity unrelated to its charitable purpose.[164] For purposes of this test, use of property bought or financed with proceeds constitutes the use of proceeds.[165] Third, no more than 2% of the proceeds from the issuance can be used to finance the costs of the issuance itself (e.g., attorney's fees, underwriter's fees, accountant's fees), and use of proceeds in this manner counts against the 5% limitation for noncharitable use.[166]

When an exempt hospital fails to abide by the foregoing restrictions, the Service can impose sanctions on the bondholders as well as the hospital. The bondholders may be required to pay tax on interest payments on the bonds retroactive to the date of issuance.[167] The exempt hospital will be treated as receiving unrelated business income in an amount equal to the fair market rental value of the bond-financed property.[168] Moreover, the exempt hospital will be precluded from deducting interest on the bond issue against the unrelated business income from the bond-financed property.[169] Ultimately, the hospital's exempt status could be placed at risk.[170] These sanctions can be avoided if certain conditions are met and (1) the bonds are immediately redeemed or (2) the facility is put to a "qualified" charitable use.[171]

Application to Hospital Joint Ventures

Exempt hospitals have little (if any) flexibility to use bond-financed property in connection with joint venture arrangements with for-profit persons. Bond-financed property may not be transferred (via sale, lease, or grant) to such a joint venture absent a redemption of the underlying bond issue.[172] Indeed, even management agreements with for-profit entities for operation of bond-financed facilities must be structured carefully to avoid any characterization that they give rise to private use of bond proceeds.[173] The Service may be more flexible, however, in permitting a joint venture to use bond-financed facilities if the venture is exclusively between 501(c)(3) exempt entities.

INTERMEDIATE SANCTIONS

Joint ventures must also be structured and operated so as to ensure that they do not violate the "Intermediate Sanctions Law," a statutory provision authorizing the Service to impose certain excise taxes whenever an exempt hospital directly or indirectly provides an "excess benefit" to a "disqualified person."[174]

General Provisions

Disqualified Persons

When scrutinizing a transaction under the Intermediate Sanctions Law, it is essential to determine whether the party receiving remuneration from the exempt hospital is a "disqualified person." Disqualified persons are identified through a two-step process.

First, the Service will identify those persons who, during the five-year period predating the transaction (the "Lookback Period"), were "in a position to exercise substantial influence over the affairs of the exempt hospital.[175] The Service has defined certain categories of persons who are *per se* disqualified persons,[176] as well as categories of persons who are *per se* not disqualified persons.[177] Determinations with respect to those persons who do not fall into either *per se* category will be made on a case-by-case basis in light of all relevant facts and circumstances.[178] Factors that the Service designates as "tending to show" that an individual had "substantial influence" over an exempt hospital include (but are not limited to) the following:

- The person founded the exempt organization.

- The person contributed over $5,000 to the exempt organization and otherwise qualifies as a "substantial contributor" under IRC § 507(d)(2).

- The person's compensation is "primarily based" on revenues derived from the activities of (1) the exempt organization as a whole or (2) a "particular department or function of the organization" that the person "controls."

- The person has or shares authority to "control" or "determine" a "substantial portion" of the exempt organization's capital expenditures, operating budget, or employee compensation.

- The person "manages" a "discrete segment or activity" of the exempt organization that "represents a substantial portion" of the exempt organization's activities, assets, income, or expenses (when compared to those of the entity as a whole).

- The person owns a "controlling interest" measured by "vote or value" in a corporation, partnership, or trust that is a disqualified person.

- The person is a "nonstock organization" directly or indirectly controlled by one or more exempt persons.[179]

Factors that the Service designates as "tending to show" that an individual has "no substantial influence" over an exempt hospital include (but are not limited to) the following:

- The person has taken a bona fide vow of poverty on behalf of a religious organization.

- The person is a contractor (e.g., attorney, accountant, investment advisor) whose "sole relationship" to the organization is the provision of "professional advice" (without decision-making authority) with respect to transactions from which such contractor "will not benefit either directly or indirectly" (aside from "customary fees" for "professional advice rendered").

- The direct supervisor of the individual is not a disqualified person.

- The person does not participate in any "management decisions" affecting (1) the exempt organization as a whole or (2) a "discrete segment or activity" of the exempt organization that "represents a substantial portion" of the exempt organization's activities, assets, income, or expenses (when compared to those of the entity as a whole).

- Any "preferential treatment" a person receives based on the size of the person's contribution is also offered to "all other donors making a comparable contribution" as part of a "solicitation intended to attract a substantial number of contributions."[180]

Second, once the Service identifies those persons who constitute disqualified persons in their own right, the Service will impute such disqualification to the family members of such disqualified persons,[181] as well as entities "35% controlled" by such disqualified persons.[182] If a corporation, partnership, or LLC is subject to the 35% control analysis and a portion of its voting stock (or profits or beneficial interests) is held by a second entity (i.e., a corporation, partnership, trust, or estate), ownership of the equity or profit interest is attributed on a pro-rata basis to the shareholders, partners, or members of the second entity, and this process is repeated until each share is traced up to an individual stakeholder (and attributed to him, his family, and his partners in any partnership).[183]

Excess Benefit. If the party receiving direct or indirect benefits from an exempt hospital is not a disqualified person, the Intermediate Sanctions Law is not implicated. If the recipient is a disqualified person, the Service will determine whether the benefit conferred on the disqualified person was an "excess" benefit. An "excess benefit" is the "amount by which the value of the economic benefit provided by" the exempt hospital to a disqualified person "exceeds the value of the consideration (including the performance of services) received for providing such benefit."[184]

Identifying the Benefits to Be Reviewed. In assessing whether the benefit conveyed by the applicable exempt organization to (or on behalf of) the disqualified person includes an "excess benefit," the Service will first identify *all* consideration and benefits conveyed to a given disqualified person by the applicable exempt organization and all organizations that it controls.[185] There are, however, two exceptions or clarifications to this general rule.

First, certain specified benefits are not included in assessing whether compensation paid is reasonable under the Intermediate Sanctions Law.[186] Exempt benefits include the following:

- Certain nontaxable fringe benefits.

- Amounts paid under reimbursement arrangements qualified under Treas. Reg. § 1.62-2(c).

- Certain economic benefits provided to volunteers; certain benefits provided to a member of an organization solely on account of the payment of a membership fee or charitable contribution of a substantial number of contributions nondisqualified persons make the same payment and receive substantially the same economic benefit.

- An economic benefit provided solely because the person is a member of a charitable class that the exempt organization intends to benefit as part of its charitable purpose.

- An economic benefit transferred to a qualified governmental unit where such transfer is "exclusively" for "public purposes."

- Payments made in accordance with certain final individual prohibited transaction exemptions issued by the Department of Labor.

Second, the Intermediate Sanctions Law does not apply to certain "fixed payments" made pursuant to an "initial" binding, written contract between the applicable exempt organization and an individual who (at least prior to execution of the contract) was not a disqualified person.[187] For purposes of the Intermediate Sanctions Law, a fixed payment ("Fixed Payment") is an amount of cash or other property specified in a contract (or determined by a formula specified in the contract) that is to be paid by or on behalf of the exempt organization or transferred for the provision of services or property similarly specified in the contract.[188] Amounts payable in connection with the following benefits are deemed "fixed" for purposes of this requirement: amounts payable under a § 401(a) qualified pension, a § 401(a) profit-sharing plan, a § 401(a) stock bonus plan, an employee benefit program satisfying certain nondiscrimination rules under the Internal Revenue Code.[189] A payment formula specified in the contract may incorporate an amount "that depends upon future specified events or contingencies" so long as no discretion is left in determining whether payment is due or the amount of such payment.[190] Substantial performance must be received by the exempt organization for the exemption to apply.[191] A contract loses the protection of this exception upon the earliest of (1) the expiration of its term, (2) the date a material change is made (including an extension or renewal of the initial term—even if through a unilateral option on the part of the person contracting with the exempt organization), or (3) the first date on which the exempt organization has the unilateral right to terminate without cause (and without incurring a substantial penalty).[192]

Valuation. Once the aggregate consideration furnished by the applicable exempt organization and its controlled entities is determined, the Service will then determine whether the consideration received in return was appropriate. The analysis varies depending upon whether compensation is purportedly for services or property.

Appropriate consideration for services is "reasonable compensation," that is, "the amount that would ordinarily be paid for like services by like enterprises (whether taxable or tax-exempt) under like circumstances.[193] The timing of the reasonableness determination varies with respect to the type of payment made. For a Fixed-Payment contract, reasonableness is determined on the date the parties enter into the compensation agreement.[194] In the case of a payment other than a Fixed Payment, reasonableness is determined based on all facts and circumstances, up to and including circumstances as of the date of payment."[195] Payment will not be deemed compensation for performance of services unless the organization documents such an intent "contemporaneous" with the economic benefit.[196] Absent such contemporaneous documentation, the payment will be considered a gratuity by the Service, increasing the risk of liability for intermediate sanctions.[197]

Appropriate consideration for property (or the right to use property) is fair market value payment, that is, payment equivalent to the price at which the property (or the right to use the property) "would change hands between a willing buyer and a willing seller, neither being under any compulsion to buy, sell, or transfer" and "both having reasonable knowledge of relevant facts."[198] The timing of the fair market value determination varies depending upon the type of property sale. If property is conveyed outright at the time of sale, the fair market value determination is made at the time of sale.[199] If the property is conveyed "subject to a substantial risk of forfeiture" and for other than a Fixed Payment, however, reasonableness is determined as of the date of payment.[200]

An applicable exempt organization can, by following certain enumerated procedures, establish a rebuttable presumption that the amount paid for services is reasonable compensation and the amount paid for property (or use of property) is fair market value.[201] The presumption, however, can only be established for Fixed Payment arrangements (or Nonfixed Payment Arrangements once the exact amount of payment or fixed formula for determining the payment amount are specified).[202] Nonetheless, once the exempt organization qualifies for the rebuttable presumption of reasonableness or fair market value, the Service must present sufficient evidence to "rebut the probative value of the comparability data relied upon by the authorized body."[203]

In order to secure the presumption of reasonableness, the relevant terms of the arrangement must be disclosed in full to an "authorized body" of the applicable exempt organization such as its governing body, a committee of its governing body (if such a committee is permitted to act on behalf of the organization under applicable state law), or others authorized by the governing body to act on its behalf by following procedures specified by the governing body in approving compensation arrangements or property transfers.[204] The authorized body must then obtain and rely upon "appropriate data as to comparability" such that the members have sufficient information to determine whether payment for services is reasonable or payment for property is fair market value.[205] Finally, the authorized body must approve the arrangement in advance of its execution and concurrently provide adequate documentation of the basis for its conclusion that the compensation for services is reasonable or sale of property is at fair market value.[206]

Direct or Indirect Provision of the Excess Benefit

A hospital can implicate the Intermediate Sanctions Law by providing an excess benefit directly or indirectly through a "controlled entity" or "intermediary."[207] A "controlled entity" is one in which the exempt hospital maintains at least a 50% interest.[208] An "intermediary" is a person who receives an economic benefit from the exempt hospital and (1) there is evidence of an understanding that the person will provide economic benefits to or for the use of a disqualified person or (2) the intermediary provides economic benefits to or for the use of a disqualified person "without a significant business purpose or exempt purpose of its own."[209]

Liability. If the Service determines that an excess benefit transaction has occurred, it can impose sanctions on both the participating disqualified persons as well as certain members of the exempt organization's management.

First, the Service can impose a 25% excise tax on the transaction for which each disqualified person receiving an excess benefit is jointly and severally liable.[210] Thereafter, the Service imposes an additional tax equal to 200% of the excess benefit if the excess benefit transaction was not "corrected" prior to the earlier of: the date on which the deficiency notice is mailed for the 25% tax or the date on which the 25% tax is assessed on the disqualified person.[211] If more than one disqualified persons received excess benefit in connection with the transaction, they are jointly and severally liable for payment of the tax.[212] The 200% tax will be abated, however, if the excess benefit transaction is corrected within 90 days thereafter.[213]

Second, in cases in which the Service imposes a 25% tax on disqualified persons, the Service generally imposes a tax of 10% of the excess benefit on any "organization manager" who "knowingly participated" in the transaction.[214] The amount collectable from organization managers in connection with the 10% tax cannot exceed $10,000 per transaction, although all managers taxed in connection with a transaction shall be joint and severally liable for taxes owed by fellow organization managers.[215] For purposes of this provision, an "organization manager" includes any officer, director, trustee (or person who, regardless of title, executes the duties or responsibilities of an officer, director, or trustee) as well as any member serving on the committee referenced in part 3.4(a)(2)(b).[216] An organization manager's actions are not "knowing" when he or she relies on a "reasoned written opinion" of an attorney, accountant, or qualified independent valuation expert acting within his or her area of expertise after disclosure of all materials facts.[217] Rather, an organization manager's participation is "knowing" only if he (1) has "actual knowledge" of sufficient facts so that (based solely upon such facts) the transaction would be an excess benefit transaction, (2) is aware that such a transaction under these circumstances may violate the provisions of federal tax law governing excess benefit transactions, and (3) either knows the transaction is an excess benefit transaction or negligently fails to make reasonable attempts to ascertain whether the transaction is an excess benefit transaction.[218]

Application to Joint Ventures. Although hospital management and the nonhospital joint venture participants bear the direct liability for any intermediate sanctions arising from joint venture transactions, the exempt hospital is best positioned to prevent such transactions from arising in the first instance. Moreover, such action is prudent on the part of the hospital in that excess benefit transactions could still give rise to impermissible private benefit or private inurement that would threaten the hospital's exempt status. Specifically, the hospital must adopt safeguards that address the risk of excess benefit transactions between the hospital and joint venture entity, the joint venture entity and third parties, and the hospital and joint venture participants. The risk of an excess benefit under each scenario will vary depending principally upon whether the hospital participates in the joint venture as an active investor (i.e., a general partner or active LLC member) or a passive investor (i.e., a limited partner, nonmanaging LLC member, or C corporation shareholder). We address the regulatory risks and appropriate safeguards under each alternative scenario.

Joint Ventures in Which the Exempt Hospital Is a General Partner or Active LLC Member. The risk of an excess benefit transaction arising from a joint venture arrangement is greatest when the exempt hospital participates as a general partner or active LLC member. First, the hospital's transactions with the joint venture itself can result in liability if more than 35% of the profit interest in the joint venture is held by disqualified persons or their family members.[219] Second, liability could also result by virtue of contracts between the joint venture and third parties (irrespective of whether the hospital is aware of the contract). As noted above, both the Service and federal courts have taken the position that when an exempt hospital participates in a joint venture as a general partner or managing LLC member, the activities of the joint venture are imputed to the hospital.[220] Thus, when a joint venture contracts with a third party, the contract could be imputed to the general partner. If that third party is a disqualified person with respect to the hospital, an excess benefit transaction could arise (even if the hospital was unaware of the existence or terms of the contract). Third, liability could arise by virtue of an exempt hospital's contract with individuals outside the joint venture arrangement altogether. If the Service does attribute the activities of the joint venture to the exempt hospital the following persons would become "disqualified persons" with respect to the hospital without ever interacting directly with the hospital:

- Persons whose compensation is "primarily based" on revenues from the joint venture (or a particular "department or function" of the joint venture) that such person controls.

- Persons who share authority to control or determine a "substantial portion" of the joint venture's capital expenditures, operating budget, or employee compensation (where they are, in turn, a "substantial portion" of the hospital's expenditures, budget, or compensation).

- Persons who "manage" joint venture activities that represent a substantial portion of the hospital's overall activities, assets, or income.

In order to minimize the threat of an excess benefit transaction under any of the foregoing scenarios, an exempt hospital should adopt a three-part strategy. First, it should ensure that it accurately values and receives appropriate consideration for property, services, or capital furnished to the joint venture itself (both during and after initial capitalization). The hospital must be particularly vigilant when disqualified persons with respect to the hospital collectively maintain 35% control in the joint venture. Therefore, the hospital should consider completing the steps necessary to establish the rebuttable presumption of reasonableness with respect to transactions involving the transfer of goods, services, or capital between the hospital and the joint venture.

Second, the exempt hospital should secure authority in the documents governing the joint venture to ensure that the hospital will receive (1) timely advance notice of contracts or transactions that the joint venture proposes to execute and that exceed a fixed dollar amount, (2) that information necessary for it to assess whether the contract poses a credible risk of an excess benefit transaction, and (3) the right to veto such an arrangement prior to execution when, in its discretion, an excess benefit transaction might result.

Third, the exempt hospital should secure authority in the documents governing the joint venture to ensure that joint venture management provide periodic updates identifying those individuals who could be considered to have "substantial influence" in connection with the joint venture. The hospital should also reserve the right to make its own independent review of joint venture records to make its own determinations on this point. If properly utilized, these disclosure and audit rights could prove invaluable to the exempt hospital in identifying individuals who become disqualified persons with respect to the hospital solely by dint of their interaction with the joint venture. Absent such disclosure, the hospital would be hard pressed to identify those individuals who might fall within this subset of its disqualified persons.

Joint Ventures in Which the Exempt Hospital Is a Limited Partner, Passive LLC Member, or C Corporation Shareholder. The risk of an excess benefit transaction arising from a joint venture arrangement is more limited when the exempt hospital participates as a limited partner, nonmanaging LLC member, or C corporation shareholder. The hospital's transactions with the joint venture itself can result in liability if more than 35% of the profit interest in the joint venture is held by disqualified persons or their family members.[221] Liability from joint venture contracts and independent hospital contracts with joint venture participants will otherwise arise only if the hospital maintains 50% control of the joint venture. If the hospital maintains such control, it is equated with the joint venture and is effectively treated as if it were an active participant. Thus, contracts between the joint venture and someone who is a disqualified person with respect to the exempt hospital could give rise to intermediate sanctions (even where the hospital is unaware of the contract or its terms). Moreover, joint venture officers, directors, employees, and managers risk becoming disqualified persons with respect to the hospital through their duties with the joint venture.

If the exempt hospital maintains less than 50% control, however, the joint venture's contracts with third parties will not give rise to an excess benefit transaction, unless the hospital affirmatively uses the joint venture as an intermediary (i.e., a conduit) to funnel excess compensation to an otherwise disqualified person. Furthermore joint venture officers, directors, employees, and managers do not risk becoming disqualified persons with respect to the hospital solely due to their duties in connection with the joint venture.

If the exempt hospital maintains less than 50% control as a limited partner, nonmanaging LLC member, or shareholder, the joint venture's provision of below-market goods or services to others are less likely to be imputed to the hospital. Similarly, those persons with substantial influence over the joint venture should not automatically become disqualified persons with respect to the hospital. Therefore, the exempt hospital can focus more specifically on its direct interactions with the joint venture and ensure that it accurately values and receives appropriate consideration for property, services or capital furnished to the joint venture itself (the hospital must be particularly vigilant when disqualified persons with respect to the hospital collectively maintain 35% control in the joint venture). Therefore, the exempt hospital should consider invoking the rebuttable presumption of reasonableness prior to the transfer of goods, services, or capital between the hospital and the joint venture. To the extent possible, the hospital should follow those procedures necessary to establish the presumption of reasonableness regarding the transaction. If the hospital maintains 50% control of the joint venture, however, it should adopt the same safeguards as appropriate for general partners and active LLC members.

ENDNOTES

1. *Redlands Surgical Services v. Commissioner*, 113 T.C. 47, 73 (1999), *aff'd* 242 F.3d 904 (9th Cir. 2001); Rev. Rul. 83-157 (Jan. 1, 1983); Rev. Rul. 69-545 (Jan. 1, 1969). The mere provision of hospital services to the paying population in a service area "does not in and of itself justify the conclusion that" a hospital is "operated exclusively for charitable purposes"; rather, "something more is required." *Sonora Community Hospital v. Commissioner*, 46 T.C. 519, 525-526 (1966), *aff'd*, 397 F.2d 814 (9th Cir. 1968); Rev. Rul. 98-15 (March 4, 1998). The Service has explicitly asserted that an organization can satisfy the community benefit standard through operation of a hospital with an emergency room open to all persons regardless of ability to pay, even where patient care is otherwise limited to patients able to pay for their care through federal or state health care programs, private insurance, or personal funds. Rev. Rul. 69-545 (Jan. 1, 1969); Rev. Rul. 83-157 (Jan. 1, 1983); Service Announcement 92-83 (May 31, 1992) ("Hospital Audit Guidelines"). When a hospital does not operate an emergency room, either due to documented excess emergency department capacity in its service area or incompatibility with the facility's clinical mission—for example, a specialized opthalmic or psychiatric hospital—it must adopt other mechanisms to ensure that it provides care for the indigent as well as the nonindigent population in its service area. Rev. Rul. 83-157 (Jan. 1, 1983). Where the amount of indigent care afforded is "de minimis" or "virtually inconsequential," exempt status will be denied. *Sonora Community Hospital*, 46 T.C. at 525-526.

2. 26 U.S.C. ("IRC") § 501(c)(3); 26 C.F.R. ("Treas. Reg.") § 1.501(c)(3)-1(a).

3. Treas. Reg. § 1.501(c)(3)-1(b)(1).

4. Treas. Reg. § 1.501(c)(3)-1(b)(2).

5. IRC § 501(c)(3); Treas. Reg. § 1.501(c)(3)-1(c).

6. Treas. Reg. § 1.501(c)(3)-1(c)(1).

7. Treas. Reg. § 1.501(c)(3)-1(c)(1).

8. IRC § 501(c)(3); Treas. Reg. §§ 1-501(c)(3)-1(c)(2), 1-501(c)(3)-1(d)(1)(ii).

9. PLR 9645018 (Aug. 9, 1996); PLR 9637050 (June 18, 1996); PLR 9231047 (May 5, 1992); PLR 9233037 (May 20, 1992); PLR 9021050 (Feb. 26, 1990).

10. GCM 39862 (Nov. 21, 1991).

11. Thomas K. Hyatt and Bruce R. Hopkins, *The Law of Tax-Exempt Healthcare Organizations* (2nd ed. 2001) ("Hyatt & Hopkins") at 60. See also PLR 39862 (Nov. 21, 1981). ("The proscription against inurement generally applies to a distinct class of private interests—typically persons who, because of their particular relationship with an organization, have opportunity to control or influence its activities.")

12. Rev. Rul. 97-21 (April 21, 1997).

13. In fact, when two parties cooperate on an ongoing basis for mutual profit, the Service and federal courts may conclude that, as a matter of law, a partnership results for tax purposes (even if formation of a partnership is contrary to the parties' intent or desire). For example, *Commissioner v. Culbertson*, 337 U.S. 733, 742 (1949).

14. An exception to this general rule arises when joint venture activity results in the generation of unrelated business income. See the section entitled "Unrelated Business Income Tax" in this chapter.

15. Michael I. Sanders, *Joint Ventures Involving Tax-Exempt Organizations* (2nd ed. 2000) ("Sanders") § 4.3. See IRC §§ 513(a), 511(a)(1); Treas. Reg. §§ 1.511-1, 1.513(a)(1). See the discussion of unrelated business income later in this chapter. There is some ambiguity as to the conditions under which the Service will deem an LLC member to be "passive" for purposes of this standard. Sanders § 4.3. Therefore, special care should be taken when relying on this provision to ensure that the exempt hospital's powers as an LLC member are sufficiently circumscribed so that it is clearly a "passive" participant in the joint venture.

16. IRC § 512(c); Rev. Rul. 98-15 (March 4, 1998) (citing *Butler v. Commissioner,* 36 T.C. 1097 (1961)); *Ward v. Commissioner,* 20 T.C. 332, 343-344 (1953), *aff'd,* 224 F.2d 547 (9th Cir. 1955).

17. See, for example, *Plumstead Theatre Society v. Commissioner,* 74 T.C. 1324, 1333-1334 (1980) (ruling that exempt organization's participation as a general partner in a limited partnership joint venture did not result in loss of exempt status where the limited partnership was operated to further a charitable purpose, the limited partners received no control over the joint venture's activities, and no private benefit or private inurement resulted from the arrangement), *aff'd* 675 F.2d 244, 244-245 (9th Cir. 1982); Rev. Rul. 98-15 (March 4, 1998). ("A 501(c)(3) organization may form and participate in a partnership, including an LLC treated as a partnership for federal income tax purposes, and meet the operational test if participation in the partnership furthers a charitable purpose and the partnership arrangement permits the exempt organization to act exclusively in furtherance of its exempt purpose and only incidentally for the benefit of the for-profit partners.")

18. Rev. Rul. 98-15 (March 4, 1998); PLR 9616005 (Dec. 19, 1995); PLR 9345057 (Aug. 20, 1993); GCM 39862 (Nov. 21, 1991); PLR 9105029 (Nov. 6, 1990); PLR 9105031 (Nov. 6, 1990); PLR 9021050 (Feb. 26, 1990); PLR 8925052 (March 28, 1989); GCM 39732 (Nov. 4, 1987); GCM 39005 (June 28, 1983).

19. *Redlands Surgical Services,* 113 T.C. at 73; Rev. Rul. 83-157 (Jan. 1, 1983); Rev. Rul. 69-545 (Jan. 1, 1969).

20. PLR 9352030 (Oct. 8, 1993). See also GCM 39732 (Nov. 4, 1987) (finding that a series of joint ventures each serves a charitable purpose when established to "provide better medical services to the public" through the establishment of new clinical services or new clinical facilities); GCM 39862 (Nov. 21, 1991). ("We recognize that there may well be legitimate purposes for joint ventures, whether analyzed under the Anti-Kickback Law or the Tax Code. These may include raising needed capital; bringing new services or a new provider to a hospital's community; sharing the risk inherent in a new activity; or pooling diverse areas of expertise.")

21. PLR 9323030 (March 16, 1993); PLR 9319044 (Feb. 18, 1993); PLR 9035072 (June 7, 1990).

22. PLR 8903060 (Oct. 25, 1988); PLR 8432014 (April 9, 1984).

23. PLR 9319044 (Feb. 18, 1993); PLR 9308034 (Nov. 30, 1992); PLR 9204048 (Oct. 30, 1991).

24. PLR 8717057 (Jan. 28, 1987).

25. GCM 39732 (Nov. 4, 1987).

26. PLR 9709014 (Nov. 26, 1996); PLR 9407022 (Nov. 22, 1993); PLR 9345057 (Aug. 20, 1993); PLR 8941006 (June 29, 1989); PLR 8946067 (Aug. 24, 1989); PLR 8936077 (June 19, 1989); PLR 8931083 (May 15, 1989); PLR 8817039 (Jan. 29, 1988); PLR 88806057 (Nov. 17, 1987); PLR 8807012 (Oct. 28, 1987); PLR 8715039 (Jan. 13, 1987); PLR 8709051 (Dec. 3, 1986); PLR 8638131 (June 30, 1986); PLR 85311069 (May 10, 1985).

27. PLR 9122061 (March 6, 1991); PLR 9105029 (Nov. 6, 1990); PLR 9024085 (March 22, 1990); PLR 9021050 (Feb. 26, 1990); PLR 8833038 (May 20, 1988); PLR 8833009 (May 19, 1988); GCM 39732 (Nov. 4, 1987); PLR 8631094 (May 7, 1986); PLR 8621059 (Feb. 25, 1986); PLR 8344099 (Aug. 5, 1983); PLR 8206093 (Nov. 10, 1981).

28. PLR 8727080 (April 10, 1987).

29. PLR 8936047 (June 13, 1989).

30. PLR 9645018 (Aug. 9, 1996); PLR 9637050 (June 18, 1996); PLR 8705089 (Nov. 7, 1986).

31. PLR 8909036 (Dec. 7, 1988).

32. PLR 8945063 (Aug. 17, 1989); PLR 8943050 (July 31, 1989); PLR 8534089 (May 31, 1985).

33. Rev. Rul. 69-464; PLR 9739041 (June 30, 1997); PLR 8940039 (July 10, 1989); PLR 8506102 (Nov. 16, 1984); PLR 8312129 (Dec. 23, 1982); PLR 8301003 (Oct. 15, 1982).

34. PLR 9518014 (Feb. 1, 1995).

35. PLR 8925052 (March 28, 1989); PLR 8915065 (Jan. 23, 1989).

36. PLR 8616005 (Dec. 19, 1995).

37. See Rev. Rul. 98-15; Rev. Rul. 69-545; PLR 9352030 (Oct. 8, 1993) (ruling that a hospital's efforts to expand and renovate its rehabilitative care facilities through a joint venture with a for-profit would not undermine its exempt status where, among other things, the partnership facility will continue to treat patients regardless of their ability to pay and will accept Medicare and Medicaid patients); PLR 9518014 (Feb. 1, 1995) (affirming that a nonprofit hospital's joint venture with a for-profit entity to furnish elder care services furthers an exempt purpose where, among other things, 4 of the 54 resident beds would be reserved for financially needy patients who will pay a reduced rate); PLR 9021050 (Feb. 26, 1990) (affirming that a hospital's joint venture with a for-profit entity to furnish elder care services furthers an exempt purpose where the joint venture facility "would "be open to the public and operated on a nondiscriminatory basis."). See also PLR 39862 (Nov. 21, 1991). ("Nearly every hospital that is an exempt organization described in section 501(c)(3) participates in the Medicare and Medicaid programs. In the usual case, doing so is a virtual requirement for exemption.")

38. FY95 CPE Text at 155-158; Unpublished PLR to Williamsburg Community Hospital (Sept. 29, 1994) ("Williamsburg Ruling"), reprinted in EOTR 1323 (Dec. 1994).

39. See FY95 CPE Text at 156 (listing "factors to consider" in determining whether an exempt hospital jeopardizes its exempt status by participation in a PHO).

40. For example, *Redlands Surgical Services*, 113 TC at 75, 77-86; *Plumstead*, 74 TC at 1333-1334; Rev. Rul. 98-15 (March 4, 1998); PLR 9645018 (Aug. 9, 1996); PLR 9616005 (Dec. 19, 1995); PLR 9345057 (Aug. 20, 1993); PLR 9308034 (Nov. 30, 1992); GCM 39862 (Nov. 21, 1991); PLR 9105029 (Nov. 6, 1990); PLR 9021050 (Feb. 26, 1990); PLR 8925052 (March 28, 1989); GCM 39732 (Nov. 4, 1987); GCM 39005 (June 28, 1983).

41. Treas. Reg. § 1.501(c)(3)-1(c)(1).

42. *Est of Hawaii v. Commissioner*, 71 T.C. 1067, 1079 (1979) (citation omitted). See also Treas. Reg. § 1.501(c)(3)-1(e) ("An organization may meet the requirements of section 501(c)(3) although it operates a trade or business as a substantial part of its activities, if the operation of such trade or business is in furtherance of the organization's exempt purpose or purposes and if the organization is not organized and operated for the primary purpose of carrying on an unrelated trade or business.").

43. *Redlands Surgical Services*, 113 T.C. at 71-72; *American Campaign Academy*, 92 T.C. at 1053, 1065 (1989). See also *Better Business Bureau of Washington, D.C. v. United States*, 326 U.S. 279, 283 (1945); *Housing Pioneers* 65 T.C. TCM 2191 (denying tax-exempt status to a general partner in a partnership providing low-income housing when a substantial purpose of the activity was to benefit commercial interests of for-profit partners), *aff'd* 58 F.3d 401 (9th Cir. 1995).

44. GCM 39005 (June 28, 1993) ("Notwithstanding an established charitable purpose, however, conflicts with charitable goals can nevertheless arise in a limited partnership situation because certain statutory obligations are imposed upon a general partner" such as "assumption of all liabilities by the general partner."); GCM 39862 (Nov. 21, 1991) ("Hospital participation in a joint venture is inconsistent with exemption, then, if . . . there is inadequate protection against financial loss by the hospital."); PLR 8638131 (June 30, 1986) (concluding that a joint venture arrangement with for-profit participants would not affect an exempt participant's exempt status where provisions in the joint venture documents resulted in "the protection of exempt assets against loss.").

45. PLR 9709014 (Nov. 26, 1996); PLR 9345057 (Aug. 20, 1993); PLR 9323030 (March 16, 1993); PLR 9319044 (Feb. 18, 1993); PLR 9308034 (Nov. 30, 1992); PLR 9122061 (March 6, 1991); PLR 9035072 (June 7, 1990); PLR 8945063 (Aug. 17, 1989); PLR 8943050 (July 31, 1989); PLR 8909036 (Dec. 7, 1988); PLR 8727080 (April 10, 1987) (tax-exempt general partner protected by insurance and indemnity agreement); PLR 8638131 (June 30, 1986) (concluding that a joint venture arrangement with for-profit participants would not affect an exempt participant's exempt status where provisions in the joint venture documents resulted in "the protection of exempt assets against loss."). See also *Plumstead Theatre Society*, 74 T.C. at 1333-1334 (ruling that a tax-exempt entity's participation as a general partner in a limited partnership advancing charitable purposes would not result in the loss of exempt status where, among other things, "[p]etitioner is not obligated for the return of any capital contribution made by the limited partners from its own funds.").

46. See Treas. Reg. § 301.7701-2 (providing that a partnership may be deemed a corporation for tax purposes if it evinces more than two of the following characteristics: centralized management, continuity of life, free transferability of interests, and limited liability); GCM 39546 (Aug. 15, 1986); PLR 8506102 (Nov. 16, 1984).

47. GCM 39862 (Nov. 21, 1991) (rejecting a joint venture in which the partnership agreement made the exempt hospital liable for any losses incurred by limited partners and required the exempt hospital to establish a "loss reserve" for such contingency); PLR 9616005 (Dec. 19, 1995) (approving exempt organization's participation in a general partnership with a for-profit entity where the exempt organization does not guarantee the venture's debt and may not borrow additional funds without the exempt entity's consent); PLR 9345057 (Aug. 20, 1993) (approving a joint venture and emphasizing that the exempt organization "is in no way obligated for the return of any capital contributions to the limited partners."); PLR 9352030 (Oct. 8, 1993) (affirming that an exempt hospital's participation in a joint venture with for-profit entities

would not affect its exempt status where, among other things, the hospital is "not required to place any" of its assets at risk other than those directly contributed to the joint venture).

48. PLR 8915065 (Jan. 23, 1989) (approving exempt entity's participation in a joint venture where the exempt entity guarantees certain joint venture debts because the guarantee was secured by sufficient collateral and required repayment at a premium); PLR 8506102 (Nov. 16, 1984) (approving a joint venture where the exempt entity guarantees a loan made to the joint venture because financial liability under the guarantee is limited in amount and required by a third-party lender, and payments made under the guarantee are subject to commercially reasonable interest backed by collateral from the limited partners).

49. GCM 39005 (June 28, 1993); GCM 39862 (Nov. 21, 1991).

50. For example, PLR 9345057 (Aug. 20, 1993); PLR 8936077 (June 19, 1989); PLR 9345057 (Aug. 20, 1993); PLR 9352030 (Oct. 8, 1993); PLR 8945063 (Aug. 17, 1989); PLR 9308034 (Nov. 30,1992). The law in some states may preclude such a provision in favor of fiduciary protections to investors, thereby necessitating that the joint venture be organized in a different state. Sanders at 137.

51. Rev. Rul. 98-15 (March 4, 1998).

52. *St. David's Health Care System*, 2003 U.S.App. LEXIS 22851 *26–*27 (5th Cir.); *Redlands Surgical Services*, 113 T.C. at 79-80; Rev. Rul. 98-15 (March 4, 1998; IRS FY 2002 CPE Text at 161). See also, for example, PLR 9637050 (June 18, 1996) (ruling that the exempt organization's participation in a joint venture with a for-profit partner would not affect its exempt status, given that the exempt organization "will retain majority ownership and control of" the joint venture, including its operational "policies and guidelines," to ensure that charitable purposes prevail when in conflict with business concerns); PLR 9709014 (Nov. 26, 1996) (ruling that the exempt organization's participation in a joint venture with a for-profit partner would not affect its exempt status, given that "management and control" of the joint venture "rests exclusively" with the exempt organization "as the sole general partner."); PLR 8638131 (June 30, 1986) (ruling that the exempt organization's participation in a joint venture with a for-profit partner would not affect its exempt status, given that the exempt entity has "effective control" of the joint venture "through its 60% general partnership interest."); PLR 8936077 (June 19, 1989) (ruling that the exempt organization's participation in a joint venture with a for-profit partner would not affect its exempt status ,given that exempt organization will hold "a majority interest" and the partnership agreement gives the exempt organization "exclusive discretion in the management and control" of the joint venture); PLR 8936077 (June 19, 1989) (ruling that the exempt organization's participation in a joint venture with a for-profit partner would not affect its exempt status, given that it will maintain "control over" the joint venture by holding "a great majority" of the joint venture equity).

53. See, for example, Rev. Rul. 98-15 (March 4, 1998); PLR 9637050 (June 18, 1996).

54. See PLR 9616005 (Dec. 19, 1995); PLR 9518014 (Feb. 1, 1995); PLR 9352030 (Oct. 8, 1993); PLR 9323030 (March 16, 1993); PLR 9319044 (Feb. 18, 1993); PLR 9318033 (Feb. 8, 1993); PLR 9308034 (Nov. 30, 1992); PLR 9105031 (Nov. 6, 1990); PLR 9105029 (Nov. 6, 1990); PLR 8945063 (Aug. 17, 1989); PLR 8943050 (July 31, 1989); PLR 8925052 (March 28, 1989); PLR 8727080 (April 10, 1987); PLR 8717057 (Jan. 28, 1987); PLR 8531069 (May 10, 1985); PLR 8206093 (Nov. 10, 1981). Indeed, the Service has previously issued guidance indicating that sufficient control could exist when the exempt participant maintained less than a 50% stake in managing the joint venture. See, for example, PLR

9122061 (March 6, 1991) (approving a joint venture in which the exempt organization held 44% of the director slots but board decisions uniformly required 66% approval for adoption and the exempt organization was responsible for day-to-day management of the facility); PLR 8909036 (Dec. 7, 1988) (approving a joint venture in which the exempt participant had only a 40% interest on the management committee and veto power over the assumption of debt by the joint venture).

55. See *St. David's Health Care System*, 2003 U.S. App. Lexis at *26–*27. ("[A]s the Government argues, there are reasons to doubt that the partnership documents provide St. David's with sufficient control" because, among other things, St. David's does not control a majority of the Board.")

56. *Redlands Surgical Services*, 113 T.C. at 80-81 (concluding that, in the absence of an outright voting majority on the part of the exempt organization, the court will "look to the binding commitments" between the nonprofit and for-profit participants "to ascertain whether other specific powers or rights conferred upon" the nonprofit entity "might compensate or mitigate for its lack of majority control.")

57. The Service has explicitly stated that it will apply the same control analysis in analyzing joint ventures to form PHOs, MSOs, and other integrated delivery systems as it does in analyzing clinical joint ventures. FY95 CPE Text at 155, 158. Although the Service initially seemed to suggest that physician representation on the board of a PHO or MSO should not exceed 20%, Service representatives have publicly abandoned this approach and conceded that the analysis to be applied in analyzing control of a PHO or MSO is identical to that applied in evaluating clinical joint ventures. Michael W. Peregrine and Bernadette M. Broccolo, PHO Tax Update, 11 EOTR 1015, 1020 (May 1995); FY95 CPE Text at 155,158.

58. *Redlands Surgical Services*, 113 T.C. at 80–81.

59. *Redlands Surgical Services*, 113 T.C. at 79–84.

60. *Redlands Surgical Services*, 113 T.C. at 84.

61. *Redlands Surgical Services*, 113 T.C. at 84.

62. *Redlands Surgical Services*, 113 T.C. at 87.

63. *St. David's Health Care System*, 2003 U.S. App. Lexis at *21, n.10, *24–*26.

64. *St. David's Health Care System*, 2003 U.S. App. Lexis at *26–*28.

65. IRC § 501(c)(3) (an organization will qualify as a tax-exempt charitable organization only if "no part of [its] net earnings . . . insures to the benefit of any private shareholder or individual."); Treas. Reg. §§ 1-501(c)(3)-1(c)(2) (providing that an organization will not qualify as a tax-exempt charitable entity if "its net earnings inure in whole or in part to the benefit of private shareholders or individuals."); 1-501(c)(3)-1(d)(1)(ii) (providing that, in order to secure exempt status, "it is necessary for an organization to establish that it is not organized or operated for the benefit of private interests").

66. *Redlands*, 113 T.C. at 74–75.

67. PLR 9645018 (Aug. 9, 1996); PLR 9637050 (June 18, 1996); PLR 9231047 (May 5, 1992); PLR 9233037 (May 20, 1992); PLR 9021050 (Feb. 26, 1990).

68. GCM 39862 (Nov. 21, 1991).

69. Hyatt & Hopkins at 60. See also PLR 39862 (Nov. 21, 1981) ("The proscription against inurement generally applies to a distinct class of private interests—typically persons who,

because of their particular relationship with an organization, have opportunity to control or influence its activities.").

70. Rev. Rul. 97-21 (April 21, 1997).

71. See, for example, Rev. Rul. 98-15 (March 4, 1998); GCM 39732 (Nov. 4, 1987); PLR 9035072 (June 7, 1990); PLR 9308034 (Nov. 30, 1992); PLR 9323030 (March 16, 1993); PLR 9318033 (Feb. 8, 1993); PLR 9345057 (Aug. 20, 1993); PLR 9645018 (Aug. 9, 1996); PLR 9637050 (June 18, 1996); PLR 9709014 (Nov. 26, 1996); PLR 9319044 (Feb. 18, 1993); PLR 8638131 (June 30, 1986); PLR 8206093 (Nov. 10, 1981); PLR 8715039 (Jan. 13, 1987); PLR 8531069 (May 10, 1985); FY95 CPE Text at 156-157; Hospital Audit Guidelines § 334.4.

72. GCM 39732 (Nov. 4, 1987); PLR 9035072 (June 7, 1990); PLR 9345057 (Aug. 20, 1993); PLR 9352030 (Oct. 8, 1993); PLR 9352030 (Oct. 8, 1993); PLR 9319044 (Feb. 18, 1993); PLR 9518014 (Feb. 1, 1995); PLR 9637050 (June 18, 1996); PLR 9645018 (Aug. 9, 1996); PLR 8945063 (Aug. 17, 1989); PLR 8909036 (Dec. 7, 1988); PLR 9021050 (Feb. 26, 1990); PLR 8727080 (April 10, 1987); PLR 8531069 (May 10, 1985); PLR 8506102 (Nov. 16, 1984); FY95 CPE text at 156–157; Hospital Audit Guidelines § 334.4.

73. *Redlands Surgical Services*, 113 T.C. at 83; PLR 9035072 (June 7, 1990); PLR 9323030 (March 16, 1993); PLR 9318033 (Feb. 8, 1993); PLR 8833038 (May 20, 1988); FY95 CPE Text at 156-157.

74. PLR 9323030 (March 16, 1993); PLR 9345057 (Aug. 20, 1993); PLR 9319044 (Feb. 18, 1993); PLR 9318033 (Feb. 8, 1993); PLR 8206093 (Nov. 10, 1981); PLR 8936077 (June 19, 1989). Hospital Audit Guidelines § 334.4.

75. PLR 9035072 (June 7, 1990); PLR 9035072 (June 7, 1990); PLR 9323030 (March 16, 1993); PLR 9345057 (Aug. 20, 1993); PLR 9637050 (June 18, 1996). Hospital Audit Guidelines § 334.4.

76. PLR 9319044 (Feb. 18, 1993) (exempt hospital has right to buy out partner's interest in joint venture after five years); PLR 8806057 (Nov. 17, 1987) (exempt hospital's participation in a joint venture with a for-profit partner will not affect its exempt status, given that the hospital "shall have the option to purchase any or all equipment, supplies, and other assets of the partnership"); Williamsburg Ruling.

77. PLR 9709014 (Nov. 26, 1996); PLR 9352030 (Oct. 8, 1993).

78. PLR 9709014 (Nov. 26, 1996).

79. Hospital Audit Guidelines § 333.4; FY95 CPE Text at 156-157; GCM 39732 (Nov. 4, 1987).

80. Hospital Audit Guidelines § 333.4; FY95 CPE Text at 156-157.

81. Hospital Audit Guidelines § 333.4; FY95 CPE Text at 156-157.

82. Hospital Audit Guidelines § 333.4; FY95 CPE Text at 156-157.

83. GCM 39862 (Nov. 21, 1991) ("One of the more troubling characteristics of the arrangements at issue is the complete lack of symmetry in upside opportunities and downside risks for the physician investors," i.e., "most of the downside risk" is borne by the exempt hospital while the physician investors receive "tremendous reward potential" with "very little downside risk."); FY95 CPE Text at 156-157.

84. PLR 9709014 (Nov. 26, 1996); PLR 9352030 (Oct. 8, 1993).

85. Rev. Rul. 98-15 (March 4, 1998); *Redlands Surgical Services*, 113 T.C. at 83.

86. *Redlands Surgical Services*, 113 T.C. at 89; PLR 9645018 (Aug. 9, 1996); PLR 8817039 (Jan.

29, 1988). Nonetheless, commercially reasonable, mutually binding covenants not to compete with the joint venture are not prohibited. PLR 9318033 (Feb. 8, 1993).

87. GCM 39862 (Nov. 21, 1991) ("[T]he private benefits conferred on the physician-investors by the instant revenue stream joint ventures are direct and substantial, not incidental. If for any reason these benefits should be found not to constitute inurement, they nonetheless exceed the bounds of prohibited private benefit). See also PLR 9231047 (May 5, 1992); PLR 9233037 (May 20, 1992).

88. Gerald M. Griffith, Refining Joint Venture Control Requirements: *St. David's v. Goliath*, EOTR (August 2002) at 255, 257.

89. An exempt hospital can create a nonprofit corporate subsidiary to participate in a joint venture activity. Moreover, if the nonprofit subsidiary qualifies for tax-exempt status, it affords the same principal benefit as a Flow-Through Entity: distributions from the joint venture will not be subject to taxation prior to or upon receipt by the exempt hospital. Nonetheless, one substantial impediment typically precludes use of such a nonprofit subsidiary in lieu of a Flow-Through Entity. The nonprofit subsidiary must establish compliance with the community benefit standard (or another basis for exemption) without reference to the charitable and other exempt activities conducted by its exempt parent. *Redlands Surgical Services*, 113 T.C. at 87 (citing *Harding Hospital v. United States*, 505 F.2d 1068 (6th Cir. 1974)). Given the limited scope of and lack of indigent care furnished in connection with many joint venture activities, this requirement may be prohibitive.

90. *Moline Properties v. Commissioner*, 319 U.S. 436, 438 (1943); *Greer v. Commissioner*, 334 F.2d 20, 23 (5th Cir. 1985); PLR 9349032 (Sept. 17, 1993); PLR 9308047 (Dec. 4, 1992); PLR 9105028 (Feb. 1, 1991); GCM 39326 (Jan. 17, 1985). For discussion of the Service's position as to when a subsidiary is deemed to be established for a legitimate business purpose and treated as a distinct entity, see GCM 35598 (Jan. 23, 1987) and GCM 39326 (Jan. 17, 1985). For a discussion of the use of a subsidiary to convey indirect private inurement, see PLR 9819046 (Feb. 11, 1998), GCM 39646 (June 30, 1987), and GCM 39598 (Jan. 23, 1987).

91. PLR 9349032 (Sept. 17, 1993); PLR 9308047 (Dec. 4, 1992).

92. IRC §§ 511(a), 512(a)(1); Treas. Reg. §§ 1.511-1, 1.511-2(a)(1)(i).

93. Treas. Reg. § 1.513-1(b).

94. Treas. Reg. § 1.513-1(b).

95. Treas. Reg. § 1.513-1(b).

96. Treas. Reg. § 1.513-1(b).

97. Treas. Reg. § 1.513-1(c).

98. Treas. Reg. § 1.513-1(d)(1).

99. Treas. Reg. § 1.513-1(d)(2).

100. Treas. Reg. § 1.513-1(d)(2); *United States v. American College of Physicians*, 475 U.S. 834, 847–848 (1986).

101. Treas. Reg. § 1.513-1(d)(3).

102. Treas. Reg. § 1.513-1(d)(3).

103. IRC §§ 512(a)(1), 512(b)(10), 512(b)(12); Treas. Reg. §§ 1.512(a)-1(a)-(c), 1.512(b)-1(g)-(h). The net operating loss deduction provided by IRC § 172 is allowed as an offset to

unrelated business taxable income. IRC § 512(b)(6). The net operating loss carryover, however, is determined without taking into account the "specific deduction" or any income or deduction that is not included under § 511 in computing unrelated business taxable income. IRC § 512(b)(6); Treas. Reg. § 1.512(b)-1(e)(1), 1.512(b)-1(g)-(h).

104. IRC § 512(b)(1)-(2); Treas. Reg. § 1.512(b)-1(a)(1), 1.512(b)-1(b).

105. IRC § 512(b)(3); Treas. Reg. § 1.512(b)-1(c)(2). If rent attributable to personal property exceeds 10% of total rent, the portion of rent attributable to such personalty will not be deemed incidental (and will therefore generate taxable income). IRC § 512(b)(3)(A)(ii); Treas. Reg. § 1.512(b)-1(c)(2)(ii)(b). If rent attributable to personal property exceeds 50% of total rent—as determined when property is first made available to the lessee under the lease—then both the rent attributable to the personalty *and the realty* will generate taxable income. IRC § 512(b)(3)(B)(i); Treas. Reg. § 1.512(b)-1(c)(2)(iii)(a). If the parties enter into separate leases for personalty and realty, the leases will be considered as one if the properties have "an integrated use." Treas. Reg. § 1.512(b)-1(c)(3)(iii). If changes are made to the lease arrangement(s) after execution, the Service will reassess compliance with the foregoing requirements. Treas. Reg. § 1.512(b)-1(c)(3)(v). Finally, rental payments for use of realty will be taxable if the exempt organization provides services for the convenience of the lessee, which are not customarily or usually furnished in connection with the rental of rooms or space for occupancy only (e.g., rent attributable to maid service as opposed to utilities or maintenance of common areas in an office complex). Treas. Reg. § 1.512(b)-1(c)(5).

106. IRC § 512(b)(5); Treas. Reg. § 1.512(b)-1(d)(1).

107. IRC § 512(b)(5); Treas. Reg. § 1.512(b)-1(d)(2). The option must be held in connection with the exempt organization's investment activities and not for sale to customers in the ordinary course of business. Treas. Reg. § 1.512(b)-1(d)(2).

108. IRC § 512(b)(8); Treas. Reg. § 1.512(b)-1(f)(3).

109. IRC § 512(b)(13).

110. IRC § 512(b)(13).

111. IRC §§ 512(b)(4), 514; Treas. Reg. § 151.512(b)-1(k), 1.514(b)-1(a). Acquisition debt includes debt incurred in acquiring or improving property. IRC § 514(c); Treas. Reg. § 1.514(c)-1(a). It also includes debt incurred after acquiring or improving the property, if the debt would not have been incurred but for the acquisition or improvement and if the need to incur such debt was reasonably foreseeable at the time of acquisition or improvement. IRC § 514(c)(1)(C); Treas. Reg. § 1.514(c)-1(a).

112. Treas. Reg. § 1.514(c)-1(a)(1)(ii).

113. IRC § 514(a)(2)-(3); Treas. Reg. § 1.514(a)-1(b). Deductions for depreciation must be made using the straight-line accounting method. Treas. Reg. § 1.514(a)-1(b)(2)(ii).

114. Treas. Reg. § 1.514(a)-1(a)(1)(v). In making this calculation, the gain or loss is multiplied against the quotient resulting from division of the highest (as opposed to the average) acquisition indebtedness on the property within the 12 months prior to disposition by the average adjusted basis for such property. Treas. Reg. § 1.514(a)-1(a)(1)(v).

115. IRC § 514(b)(1)(A); Treas. Reg. § 1.514(b)-1(b)(1). In identifying the proportion of property "use" devoted to exempt purposes, the Service will look at the amount of time during which the property is used for exempt purposes in contrast to the amount of time during

which the property is used for other purposes. Treas. Reg. § 1.514(b)-1(b)(1)(ii). The Service will also look at the portion of property used for exempt purposes in comparison to the proportion of property used for other purposes. Treas. Reg. § 1.514(b)-1(b)(1)(ii). Use by related entities shall be considered when determining whether property is devoted to research activities. Treas. Reg. § 1.514(b)-1(b)(6).

116. IRC § 514(b)(1)(B); Treas. Reg. § 1.514(b)-1(b)(2). Nonetheless, any gain on the disposition of such property that is not recognized as unrelated business taxable income must be included as income derived from debt financed property. Treas. Reg. § 1.514(b)-1(b)(2).

117. IRC § 514(b)(1)(C); Treas. Reg. § 1.514(b)-1(b)(4). Research conducted by a related organization shall be considered when determining whether property is devoted to research activities. IRC § 514(b)(1)(C); Treas. Reg. § 1.514(b)-1(b)(6).

118. IRC § 514(b)(1); Treas. Reg. § 1.514(b)-1(c)(1).

119. IRC § 514(b)(2); Treas. Reg. § 1.514(b)-1(c)(2).

120. IRC § 514(b)(3); Treas. Reg. § 1.514(b)-1(d).

121. IRC § 514(c)(2); Treas. Reg. § 1.514(c)-1(b)(3).

122. IRC § 512(c); Treas. Reg. § 1.512(c)-1. See also *Service Bolt & Nut Co. v. Commissioner*, 724 F.2d 519, 522-523 (6th Cir. 1983); Rev. Rul. 79-222 (Jan. 1, 1979); PLR 9703026 (Oct. 29, 1996). Income to a 501(c)(3) organization from an S corporation is automatically deemed to be unrelated business income. IRC § 512(e).

123. Treas. Reg. § 1.513-1(d)(1).

124. Treas. Reg. § 1.513-1(d)(2); *American College of Physicians*, 475 U.S. at 847-848.

125. Treas. Reg. § 1.513-1(d)(3).

126. Treas. Reg. § 1.513-1(d)(3).

127. IRC § 513(a); Treas. Reg. § 1.513-1(e)(2). There has been some debate as to whether staff physicians in private practice are "members" of a hospital. Compare *St. Luke's Hospital of Kansas City*, 494 F. Supp. 85, 92-93 (W.D. Mo. 1980) (stating that physicians on a hospital's medical staff are "members" within the meaning of IRC § 513(a)(2)) with Rev. Rul. 85-109 (stating that the Service disagrees with and will not abide by the court's conclusion in *St. Luke's Hospital of Kansas City v. U.S.* that staff physicians in private practice are "members" of the hospital for purposes of IRC § 513).

128. Rev. Rul. 68-376; PLR 8246018 (Aug. 20, 1982); PLR 8206093 (Nov. 10, 1981). See also *Carle Foundation v. United States*, 611 F.2d 1192, 1199 (7th Cir. 1979) (describing the foregoing rulings).

129. Rev. Rul. 69-268; Rev. Rul. 69-269.

130. Hyatt & Hopkins at § 24.5.

131. PLR 8531069 (May 10, 1985); PLR 8638131 (June 30, 1986); PLR 8709051 (Dec. 3, 1986); PLR 8715039 (Jan. 13, 1987); PLR 8807012 (Oct. 28, 1987); PLR 8806057 (Nov. 17, 1987); PLR 8817039 (Jan. 29, 1988); PLR 8936077 (June 19, 1989); PLR 8941006 (June 29, 1989); PLR 8946067 (Aug. 24, 1989); PLR 9204048 (Oct. 30, 1991); PLR 9407022 (Nov. 22, 1993); PLR 9709014 (Nov. 26, 1996).

132. PLR 9122061 (March 6, 1991); PLR 9105029 (Nov. 6, 1990); PLR 8833038 (May 20, 1988).

133. PLR 8925052 (March 28, 1989).

134. PLR 8717057 (Jan. 28, 1987).

135. PLR 9518014 (Feb. 1, 1995).

136. PLR 8727080 (April 10, 1987).

137. PLR 9318033 (Feb. 8, 1993); PLR 9308034 (Nov. 30, 1992).

138. PLR 9319044 (Feb. 18, 1993).

139. PLR 8903060 (Oct. 25, 1988); PLR 8432014 (April 9, 1984).

140. PLR 9035072 (June 7, 1990).

141. PLR 9323030 (March 16, 1993).

142. PLR 9352030 (Oct. 8, 1993).

143. PLR 8909036 (Dec. 7, 1988).

144. 8945063 (Aug. 17, 1989); PLR 8943050 (July 31, 1989); PLR 8934089 (May 31, 1985).

145. PLR 9645018 (Aug. 9, 1996); PLR 9637050 (June 18, 1996).

146. PLR 9722042 (March 7, 1997); PLR 9721031 (Feb. 26, 1997); PLR 9714011 (Dec. 24, 1996); PLR 9651047 (Sept. 24, 1996).

147. PLR 9739036 (June 30, 1997). See also PLR 9837031 (June 15, 1988).

148. FY95 CPE Text at 159-160.

149. FY95 CPE Text at 159-160.

150. FY95 CPE Text at 159-160.

151. IRC §§ 512(a)(1), 512(b)(10), 512(b)(12); Treas. Reg. §§ 1.512(a)-1(a)-(c), 1.512(b)-1(g)-(h).

152. IRC § 512(b)(6).

153. IRC § 512(b)(6); Treas. Reg. § 1.512(b)-1(e)(1), 1.512(b)-1(g)-(h).

154. See *supra* part 3.2(a)(2)(b).

155. PLR 9349032 (Sept. 17, 1993); PLR 9308047 (Dec. 4, 1992).

156. IRC § 512(b)(13). This will be true even when the joint venture is structured as a Flow-Through Entity.

157. IRC § 512(b)(13).

158. For purposes of this section, we assume that tax-exempt bonds issued by an exempt hospital qualify for exemption on the basis that they are 501(c)(3) bonds.

159. IRC § 103(a); Treas. Reg. § 1.145-1(a).

160. FY99 CPE at 155.

161. IRC §§ 103(b), 141(e)(1)(G); Treas. Reg. § 1.145-1(a).

162. IRC § 145(a)(1); Treas. Reg. § 1.145-2(b)(3). Portions of a facility owned and used by an exempt hospital in furtherance of its charitable purpose may also be used by nonexempt persons, but only that portion of a "mixed-use facility" owned and used by the hospital may be financed with exempt funds. PLR 9125050 (March 29, 1991); PLR 8827065 (April 14, 1988). The Service has recognized a number of accounting methods to apportion the exempt and nonexempt use of the facility to identify the portion which may be financed

with tax exempt bonds (e.g., allocation by square foot, fair market value, or per procedure). See PLR 9125050 (March 29, 1991); PLR 8827065 (April 14, 1988).

163. IRC § 145(a)(2); Treas. Reg. § 1.145-2(b)(1)-(2). For purposes of this requirement, "net proceeds" are aggregate proceeds from the bond issuance (including proceeds used to pay for the cost of the bond issuance) less amounts maintained in a limited reserve fund. IRC § 148(d). The average maturity on an issue of 501(c)(3) bonds generally may not exceed 120% of the expected economic life of the facilities financed with proceeds from the issue. IRC § 147(b). Finally, there are restrictions on tax arbitrage of bond proceeds as well as procedural requirements for registering and securing public approval for the issuance of such bonds. See IRC §§ 147(f), 148, 149(a), 149(e).

164. IRC § 145(a)(2); Treas. Reg. § 1.145-2(b)(1)-(2).

165. Treas. Reg. § 1.141-3(a).

166. IRC § 147(g)(1); Treas. Reg. § 1.145-2.

167. IRC § 103(b). Such interest will also likely be factored into computation of the bondholder's alternative minimum tax. IRC § 57.

168. IRC § 150(b)(3)(A).

169. IRC § 150(b)(3)(B).

170. FY99 CPE at 157.

171. Treas. Reg. §§ 1.141-12, 1.150-4; Rev. Proc. 93-17 (Feb. 19, 1993).

172. Treas. Reg. § 1.145-2(b) (cross referencing Treas. Reg. § 1.141-3(a)-(b)); IR 90-60 (Jan. 2, 1990).

173. Treas. Reg. § 1.145-2(b) (cross referencing Treas. Reg. § 1.141-3(a)-(b)); Rev. Proc. 97-13 (Jan. 10, 1997).

174. IRC § 4958(a)-(b). As noted above, for purposes of this chapter, we assume that the hospital's exempt status is predicated upon § 501(c)(3) of the Code. If not, the Intermediate Sanctions Law may not apply. IRC § 4958(e); Treas. Reg. § 53.4958-2(a). We also note that a hospital relinquishing exempt designation remains subject to the Intermediate Sanctions Law for transactions occurring in the ensuing five years.

175. IRC § 53.4958(f)(1)(A); Treas. Reg. § 53.4958-3(a). When a transaction involves multiple affiliated exempt organizations, the determination as to whether one is a "disqualified person" must be made separately with respect to each entity. Treas. Reg. § 53.4958-3(f). Nonetheless, a person may be a "disqualified person" with respect to more than one of the affiliated entities. Treas. Reg. § 53.4958-3(f).

176. Persons who meet any of the following requirements during the Lookback Period for the transaction in question are deemed, *per se*, to be "disqualified persons" under the Intermediate Sanctions Law: (1) voting members of the exempt organization's governing authority, and (2) persons who, regardless of title, have ultimate responsibility for implementing the decisions of the governing body or supervising the management, administration, or operation of the organization or managing its finances. Treas. Reg. § 53.4958-3(c). The president, chief executive officer, chief operating officer, treasurer, and chief financial officer are deemed to have such responsibility unless they demonstrate otherwise. Treas. Reg. § 53.4958-3(c). Any person with a "material financial interest in a provider-

sponsored organization ("PSO") in which a tax-exempt hospital participates is deemed a disqualified person with respect to the hospital. Treas. Reg. § 53.4958-3(c).

177. Persons deemed, *per se, not* to be "disqualified persons" under the Intermediate Sanctions Law include: (1) 501(c)(3) organizations, (2) 501(c)(4) organizations under certain circumstances, and (3) certain employees who receive economic benefits from the exempt organization which, in aggregate, are less than the amount designated by the Service for qualification as a "highly compensated" employee.

178. Treas. Reg. § 53.4958-3(a).

179. Treas. Reg. § 53.4958-3(e)(2).

180. Treas. Reg. § 53.4958-3(e)(3).

181. IRC § 4958(f); Treas. Reg. § 53.4958-3(b). A disqualified person's "family" is limited to his or her spouse, brothers or sisters (by whole or half blood), spouses of brother or sisters (by whole or half blood), ancestors, children (or their spouses), grandchildren (or their spouses), and great grandchildren (or their spouses).

182. Determination as to whether such control exists varies depending upon the type of organization involved. For a corporation, disqualified persons (including their families) must hold 35% of the "combined voting power" (i.e., 35% of the "voting stock") of the corporation. IRC § 4956(f)(3)(A)(i); Treas. Reg. § 53.4958-3(b)(2). For a partnership, disqualified persons (including their families) must hold 35% of the profit interest. IRC § 4956(f)(3)(A)(ii); Treas. Reg. § 53.4958-3(b)(2). For a trust or estate, disqualified persons (including their families) must hold 35% of the beneficial interest. IRC § 4956(f)(3)(A)(iii); Treas. Reg. § 53.4958-3(b)(2).

183. IRC § 4958(f)(3)(B); Treas. Reg. § 53.4958-3(b)(2)(iii).

184. IRC § 4958(c)(1); Treas. Reg. §§ 53.4958-1(b), 53.4958-4(a).

185. Treas. Reg. § 53.4958-4(a)(1).

186. Treas. Reg. § 53.4958-4(a)(4).

187. Treas. Reg. §§ 53.4958-4(a)(3)(i), 53.4958-4(a)(3)(iii).

188. Treas. Reg. § 53.4958-4(a)(3)(ii)(A).

189. Treas. Reg. § 53.4958-4(a)(3)(ii)(B).

190. Treas. Reg. § 53.4958-4(a)(3)(ii)(A).

191. Treas. Reg. § 53.4958-4(a)(3)(iv).

192. Treas. Reg. § 53.4958-4(a)(3)(v).

193. Treas. Reg. § 53.4958-4(b)(1)(ii)(A). In determining reasonableness, the Service will abide by the standards used to determine whether compensation is "reasonable" for purposes of qualifying as an itemized deduction for federal income tax. Treas. Reg. § 53.4958-4(b)(1)(ii)(A). Again, when assessing the reasonableness of compensation, the Service reviews the aggregate of *all* compensation and benefits not explicitly exempted above paid by the applicable exempt organization and those organizations it controls. Treas. Reg. § 53.4958-4(b)(1)(ii)(B). The fact that compensation is subject to a cap "is a relevant factor in determining the reasonableness of compensation." Treas. Reg. § 53.4958-4(b)(1)(ii)(A).

194. Treas. Reg. § 53.4958-4(b)(2)(i). The one exception to this rule occurs when substantial performance is not made on the contract. In such cases, the reasonableness determination will be made in the same manner as with a non-Fixed Payment. Treas. Reg. § 53.4958-4(b)(2)(i). In determining the date of contract for purposes of making the reasonableness determination, a contract becomes a wholly new contract (necessitating a new reasonableness determination) as of the earliest of (1) the expiration of its term, (2) the date a material change is made (including an extension or renewal of the initial term—even if through a unilateral option on the part of the person contracting with the exempt organization), or (3) the first date on which the exempt organization has the unilateral right to terminate without cause (and without incurring a substantial penalty). Treas. Reg. § 53.4958-4(a)(3)(v).

195. Treas. Reg. § 53.4958-4(b)(2)(i).

196. Treas. Reg. § 53.4958-4(c)(1). Contemporaneous documentation can include Forms W-2 or 1099 filed by the Exempt Organization, tax returns filed by the disqualified person, an approved written employment agreement executed no later than the date of initial payment, certain documentation indicating that an Authorized Body approved the transaction on or before the date of transfer, etc. Treas. Reg. § 53.4958-4(c)(3)(ii). The sole exceptions to the contemporaneous documentation requirement are (1) for benefits excluded from the disqualified person's gross income under chapter 1, subtitle A of the Internal Revenue Code (e.g., employer-provided health benefits, contributions to a pension, profit-sharing, or stock bonus plan qualified under IRC § 401(a)), and (2) cases in which the applicable tax exempt organization demonstrates that its failure to maintain appropriate documentation was due to "reasonable cause" (i.e., there are certain mitigating factors or factors beyond the organization's control). Treas. Reg. §§ 53.4958-4(c)(3)(i)(B), 53.4958-4(c)(1). Such benefits are still included in making the reasonableness determination unless they qualify as an Excluded Benefit .

197. Treas. Reg. § 53.4958-4(c)(1).

198. Treas. Reg. § 53.4958-4(b)(1)(i).

199. Treas. Reg. § 53.4958-4(b)(1)(i). In determining the date of contract for purposes of making the reasonableness determination, a contract becomes a wholly new contract (necessitating a new reasonableness determination) as of the earliest of (1) the expiration of its term, (2) the date a material change is made (including an extension or renewal of the initial term—even if through a unilateral option on the part of the person contracting with the exempt organization), or (3) the first date on which the exempt organization has the unilateral right to terminate without cause (and without incurring a substantial penalty). Treas. Reg. § 53.4958-4(a)(3)(v).

200. Treas. Reg. § 53.4958-4(b)(1)(i).

201. Treas. Reg. § 53.4958-6(a). Failure to obtain the rebuttable presumption of reasonableness does not, however, raise an inference that the transaction involves an excess benefit.

202. Treas. Reg. § 53.4958-6(d)(1). Employment arrangements subject to a cap will be treated as Fixed Payment arrangements with respect to the capped amount. Treas. Reg. § 53.4958-6(d)(2).

203. Treas. Reg. § 53.4958-6(b).

204. Treas. Reg. §§ 53.4958-6(a)(1), 53.4958-6(c)(1)(i). This body must be composed entirely of persons with no conflict of interest relating to the transaction reviewed. Treas. Reg. § 53.4958-6(c)(1)(i).

205. Treas. Reg. § 53.4958-6(a)(2). Relevant information for evaluating compensation arrangements might include compensation paid by similarly situated organizations for similar services, the availability of similar services in the exempt organization's geographic area, current compensation surveys compiled by independent firms, written offers from similar institutions competing for the services of the disqualified person. Treas. Reg. § 53.4958-6(c)(2)(i). Alternative means of defining comparability data apply for organizations with annual gross receipts of less than $1 million. Treas. Reg. § 53.4958-6(c)(2)(ii). Relevant information for evaluating a property sale might include independent appraisals or offers received through competitive and open bidding. Treas. Reg. § 53.4958-6(c)(2)(i). Alternative means of defining comparability data apply for organizations with annual gross receipts of less than $1 million. Treas. Reg. § 53.4958-6(c)(2)(ii).

206. Treas. Reg. § 53.4958-6(a)(3). Such documentation must include the terms of the transaction; the date on which it was approved; the members of the committee present during debate on the transaction; members voting on the transaction; the comparability data obtained and relied upon; the manner in which such comparability data was obtained; the basis for any fair market value or reasonable compensation range set by the authorized body, which is distinct from that in the comparability data; any actions taken by a person who is otherwise a member of the authorized body but who had a conflict of interest with respect to the transaction. Treas. Reg. § 53.4958-6(a)(3). The Service has published two "checklists" for adequate documentation. See FY02 CPE at 327-332. The documentation will be deemed concurrent with the transaction before the later of the next meeting of the authorized body or 60 days after final action by the governing body on the transaction. Treas. Reg. § 53.4958-6(a)(3).

207. IRC § 4958(c)(1); Treas. Reg. § 53.4958-4(a)(2).

208. Treas. Reg. § 53.4958-4(a)(2)(ii). The hospital will be deemed to own a 50% interest in an entity if it owns 50% of the stock vote or value (in the case of a controlled corporation), owns 50% of the profit or capital interests (in the case of a controlled partnership), "directly or indirectly" controls 50% of the directors or trustees (in the case of a controlled nonstock entity), or owns more than 50% of the beneficial interest (in the case of any other entity). An individual serving as a director or trustee is a "representative" of the exempt organization if he or she acts as a trustee, director, agent, or employee of the exempt organization. Treas. Reg. § 53.4958-4(a)(2)(ii)(B)(iii).

209. Treas. Reg. § 53.4958-4(a)(2)(iii).

210. IRC §§ 4958(a)(1), 4958(d)(1); Treas. Reg. §§ 53.4958-1(c)(1), 53.4958-1(c)(2)(i).

211. IRC § 4958(b); Treas. Reg. § 53.4958-1(c)(2)(ii). "An excess benefit transaction is corrected by undoing the excess benefit to the extent possible, and taking any additional measures necessary to place the applicable tax exempt organization involved in the excess benefit transaction in a financial position not worse than that in which it would be if the disqualified person were dealing under the highest fiduciary standards." IRC § 4958(f)(6); Treas. Reg. § 53.4958-7(a). See Treas. Reg. § 53.4958-(7) for greater detail on appropriate means for "correction."

212. IRC § 4958(d)(1); Treas. Reg. § 53.4958-1(d)(8).

213. Treas. Reg. § 53.4958-1(c)(2)(iii).

214. IRC § 4958(a)(2); Treas. Reg. § 53.4958-1(d)(1). For purposes of this requirement, "participation" includes affirmative action as well as silence or inaction when the organization

manager is under a duty to act. Treas. Reg. § 53.4958-1(d)(3). Affirmative opposition to a transaction by an organization manager, consistent with the fulfillment of his or her responsibilities, does not constitute "participation." Treas. Reg. § 53.4958-1(d)(1).

215. IRC § 4958(d); Treas. Reg. § 53.4958-1(d)(7)-(8).

216. IRC § 4958(f)(2); Treas. Reg. § 53.4958-1(d)(2). An "officer" includes anyone designated as such under the exempt organization's governing documents as well as anyone who "regularly exercises general authority to make [not just recommend] administrative or policy decisions on behalf of the organization." Treas. Reg. § 53.4958-1(d)(2). A contractor acting solely in the capacity of an accountant, attorney, investment manager, or advisor is not an officer. Treas. Reg. § 53.4958-1(d)(2).

217. Treas. Reg. § 53.4958-1(d)(4)(iii). A "reasoned written opinion" may not summarily recite the applicable facts and a conclusion. Treas. Reg. § 53.4958-1(d)(4)(iii). Rather, it must cite the applicable law and expressly apply it to the relevant facts. Treas. Reg. § 53.4958-1(d)(4)(iii).

218. Treas. Reg. § 53.4958-1(d)(4)(i). The sole exception to the 10% tax applies when the organization manager's participation in the transaction was (1) "not willful" and (2) due to "reasonable cause." Treas. Reg. § 53.4958-1(d)(2). A manager's actions are not willful if he "does not know" the transaction at issue is an excess benefit transaction. Treas. Reg. § 53.4958-1(d)(5). His or her participation shall be deemed due to "reasonable cause" if he or she has used "ordinary business care and prudence" in reviewing the transaction. Treas. Reg. § 53.4958-1(d)(5).

219. IRC § 4958(f)(3); Treas. Reg. 53.4958-3(b)(2)(i)(B).

220. See note 16 in this handbook and accompanying text.

221. IRC § 4958(f)(3); Treas. Reg. § 53.4958-3(b)(2)(i)(B).

CHAPTER 4

Federal Antitrust Laws Governing Hospital Joint Ventures

INTRODUCTION

General Provisions

Hospital joint ventures can, under certain conditions, raise compliance concerns under federal antitrust laws. The most pertinent antitrust authorities are the Sherman Antitrust Act, the Clayton Antitrust Act, the Federal Trade Commission Act, the National Cooperative Research and Production Act ("NCRPA"), and the Hart-Scott-Rodino Antitrust Improvements Act of 1976 ("HSRA").[1] Each such measure is briefly described below.

The Sherman Act imposes two substantive restrictions. Section 1 of the Sherman Act prohibits any contract, combination, or conspiracy that constitutes an unreasonable restraint on interstate or foreign commerce.[2] Section 2 of the Sherman Act prohibits monopolization as well as attempts to monopolize or conspiracies to monopolize in interstate or foreign commerce.[3] Corporations violating either provision are subject to a criminal fine of up to the greatest of $10 million, twice the corporation's pecuniary gain, or twice the victims' pecuniary loss.[4] Individuals are subject to three years' imprisonment and a criminal fine amounting to the greatest of $350,000, twice the resulting pecuniary gain, or twice the resulting pecuniary loss.[5] The government may also proceed with a civil action in response to a violation of either section.[6]

Section 7 of the Clayton Act prohibits mergers, acquisitions, and certain joint ventures that may serve to "substantially" lessen competition or to "tend to create a monopoly."[7] Upon detecting a violation of § 7, the government can secure an administrative cease and desist order, injunction, divestiture order, or conduct order.[8] Private parties and the federal government can also secure treble damages and injunctive relief for injuries suffered due to a violation of § 7.[9]

The Federal Trade Commission Act authorizes the Federal Trade Commission ("FTC") to prevent "unfair methods of competition" in interstate and foreign commerce, including violation of the Sherman and Clayton Acts.[10] The FTC is empowered to impose a cease and desist order to stop such practices.[11] The FTC, however, lacks jurisdiction over most nonprofit entities, with the principal exception being nonprofit entities that furnish substantial pecuniary benefits to their members or their members' businesses (e.g., professional societies).[12]

NCRPA provides specific standards and limitations on liability associated with qualified joint ventures for the production of items, the furnishing of services, and certain research and development activities.[13] Specifically, the NCRPA provides that such joint ventures are not *per se* illegal, and must be evaluated through the flexible "rule of reason" standard described below.[14] Anticompetitive dealings between participants in a qualified joint venture will not be protected, however, unless those dealings are reasonably related to the joint venture itself.[15] If the joint venture makes certain disclosures to DOJ/FTC regarding the purpose of and participants in the joint venture, private and state antitrust claims will be limited to actual damages, attorneys fees, costs, and interest.[16]

HSRA mandates that, under certain circumstances, those forming a joint venture file advance written notice of the transaction and submit to prior review by DOJ/FTC.[17] Creation of a joint venture in the form of a partnership or limited partnership will not necessitate an HSR filing.[18] Formation of a joint venture as an LLC will not necessitate an HSR filing unless two or more separately controlled businesses are contributed to the LLC upon formation and at least one party retains a 50% or greater interest in the joint venture.[19] Formation of a joint venture as a corporation (or an LLC involving the contribution of two or more businesses under the 50% control of at least one party), will implicate the Act if either of the following occurs:

- The capital and credit extended by joint venture participants to the joint venture exceeds $200 million; or

- The capital and credit extended by joint venture participants to the joint venture exceeds $50 million, and either:

  - The joint venture will have $100 million or more in assets and two or more joint venture investors maintain $10 million in assets or annual net sales; or

  - The joint venture will have $10 million or more in assets, one of the investors maintains $10 million in assets or annual net sales, and a second investor maintains $100 million or more in net sales or total assets.[20]

APPLICATION TO HOSPITAL JOINT VENTURES

Although hospitals that are run as an instrumentality of a state or local government can qualify for immunity under these laws pursuant to the state action doctrine, the doctrine provides little practical protection to hospital joint ventures, given that (1) most hospitals do not qualify as state instrumentalities and (2) even those hospitals that do so qualify are protected from federal antitrust law only in connection with activities that are an authorized implementation of a clearly articulated state policy.[21] Thus, those developing hospital joint ventures must be mindful of applicable federal antitrust laws.

Hospital joint ventures typically fall into either of two categories: (1) joint ventures to furnish clinical services or acquire clinical facilities or equipment ("Clinical Joint Ventures") or (2) provider networks (including physician hospital organizations) for the furnishing of clinical services ("Network Arrangements"). These two types of joint ventures raise distinct antitrust concerns and are therefore addressed separately below. Thereafter, we address concerns relating to the sharing of information between potential competitors, sharing that can arise in the operation of either category of joint venture.

Clinical Joint Ventures

Overview

DOJ/FTC recognize that Clinical Joint Ventures involving actual or potential competitors will most often give rise to overall procompetitive efficiencies benefiting consumers (e.g., economies of scale, provision of new technologies not otherwise affordable, combinations of complementary resources, or expertise).[22] Indeed, they have not yet challenged a Clinical Joint Venture on antitrust grounds. Nonetheless, those forming or operating a Clinical Joint Venture should be aware that the arrangement might give rise to antitrust concerns if two or more participants are actual or potential competitors in a given market. A firm is deemed to be a "potential competitor" of a second firm if (1) it is "reasonably probable" that the firm would enter the same product and geographic market as the second firm, in the absence of the relevant agreement or (2) "competitively significant decisions by actual competitors" in an existing product and geographic market are "constrained by concerns" that "anticompetitive conduct" would likely induce the firm to enter the market.[23]

Under such circumstances, DOJ/FTC might inquire whether the joint venture serves as a vehicle through which potential or actual competitors could collude to undermine competition. Specifically, if the joint venture is formed to compete in a market in which the joint venture participants already have a presence, the government might inquire whether the would-be competitors could achieve such collective market power through the joint venture that they could act in concert internally, or with one or more remaining competitors, to raise prices, reduce output, or reduce quality.[24] Alternatively, if the joint venture participates in markets distinct from those in which the participants compete, the government might inquire whether the joint venture might serve as a forum in which the participants could collude to undermine competition in the markets in which they do compete.[25]

Review Process

Given these countervailing concerns, when reviewing a Clinical Joint Venture between actual or potential competitors, DOJ/FTC will assess whether (1) the venture is likely to promote or impede competition in the markets it serves and (2) all agreements between the competitors in connection with the joint venture relating to price, output, or quality of items or services are "reasonably necessary" to achieve procompetitive efficiencies through joint venture integration.[26] This is referred to as the "rule of reason" analysis.[27] It can best be understood as a four-step process. Each step is addressed, in turn, below.

Identifying the Market. First, DOJ/FTC will define those product and geographic markets in which the joint venture will compete (e.g., provision of MRI services in a given town). The relevant product market comprises the array of goods or services that a given consumer (e.g., physician or patient) would consider as a substitute for services to be furnished through the joint venture.[28] For purposes of this analysis, DOJ/FTC (1) assume that the joint venture has a monopoly for each specific item or service it furnishes, (2) assume that the joint venture imposes a small but significant and nontransitory price increase (typically 5%) for its items and services, and (3) identify those items or services to which consumers (e.g., physicians or patients) would turn to as an alternative in the wake of the joint venture's price increase.[29] The relevant geographic market is the smallest geographic area in which a monopolist within the area could impose a small but significant and nontransitory price increase in the product market without consumers turning to producers who are located outside the given area.[30]

Assessing the Potential for Anticompetitive Collusion in the Relevant Market. Second, DOJ/FTC will assess the potential for anticompetitive collusion in the given product and geographic market ("Market") as a result of the joint venture.[31] This involves a review of four principal factors: (1) the share of the Market actually/likely maintained by the joint venture, (2) the share of the Market maintained independently by joint venture participants, (3) the overall level of supplier concentration within the Market, and (4) the relative barriers to entry into the Market by new competitors.[32]

The greater the share of the Market maintained by the joint venture, the more readily it can reduce aggregate output within the Market to support a price increase.[33] This concern is particularly pronounced if (1) competitors in the Market will be terminating competition in favor of collaboration through the joint venture, and (2) the items or services previously furnished on an independent basis by the joint venture participants were viewed as closer substitutes for each other than for other products within the Market.[34] DOJ/FTC maintain that, under such circumstances, the joint venture participants placed more significant competitive restraints on each other prior to the joint venture because consumers saw them as more fungible substitutes and would readily switch to the second competitor if the first imposed a price increase.[35]

The possibility of anticompetitive behavior exists even if the joint venture participants purport to remain in competition with the joint venture (and each other) in a given Market. The greater the share of the Market maintained independently by joint venture participants ostensibly remaining in competition within the Market, the more effectively they can collude with the joint venture to reduce output and increase price.[36] In determining the threat of anticompetitive collusion posed by a joint venture (whether between the joint venture and joint venture participants or between some combination of them and the remaining competitors in the Market), DOJ/FTC will consider whether the following additional factors exist to facilitate collusion: (1) availability of information regarding market conditions, individual transactions, and individual competitors so as to monitor compliance among colluding parties and punish deviations from agreed output levels allotted to each, (2) product homogeneity within the Market, (3) previous collusion within the Market, and (4) previous collusion within the same product market in a different geographic market.[37]

DOJ/FTC's concern with the potential anticompetitive effects of a joint venture will vary in proportion to the level of Market concentration. The greater the level of concentration within the Market, the more readily the venture could collude with one or more competitors within the Market to effectively reduce output and increase prices.[38] Conversely, DOJ/FTC's concern that a joint venture might facilitate anticompetitive behavior (whether by amassing market power in its own right or colluding with joint venture participants or other ostensible competitors) will be substantially ameliorated when the Market is of such a nature that new firms could cost-effectively enter into competition with sufficient speed and in sufficient volume to punish a substantial price increase.[39]   DOJ/FTC believe such a dynamic would deter a firm with market power from raising prices through reduced output and would punish competitors who enacted such increases.[40]

Assessing the Likelihood of Anticompetitive Collusion Third, if the Market is of such a nature that anticompetitive collusion might be feasible through the joint venture, DOJ/FTC will examine the specifics of the venture to assess whether it is structured in a manner that would encourage, minimize, or deter collusion among the participants.[41] This analysis will focus on several factors, including the following:

- **Exclusivity:** The extent to which the joint venture participants are likely to continue competing independently in the Market outside the joint venture. Competitiveness is promoted if joint venture participants competing in the Market continue to do so after formation of the joint venture.[42]

- **Duration:** The duration of the joint venture. Competitiveness is generally reduced as the proposed duration of the joint venture is increased.[43]

- **Assets:** The extent to which the joint venture participants are required to contribute assets to the joint venture which thereby impede their further effective competition in the markets in which the joint venture operates. Competitiveness is reduced when participants are required to contribute such specialized assets to the joint venture, particularly if the assets cannot be readily replaced.[44]

- **Extent of Joint Venture Investment:** The extent (both in size and nature) of each participant's interest in the joint venture. Competitiveness is reduced to the extent that those in a position to compete with the joint venture maintain a substantial share in the arrangement or in another joint venture participant with a substantial share in the arrangement.[45]

- **Control over Joint Venture Decisions:** The extent to which joint venture participants are able to exercise significant control over daily joint venture operations. Competitiveness is reduced to the extent that joint venture participants gain greater control over competitively significant decisions such as the venture's output and pricing strategies.[46]

- **Likelihood of Anticompetitive Information Sharing:** The extent to which competitively-sensitive information concerning markets affected by collaboration would be disclosed. Competitiveness is promoted to the extent that the amount of competitively-sensitive information disseminated to joint venture participants is reduced through appropriate safeguards.[47]

Balancing Potential Anticompetitive Effects Against Likely Efficiencies
If DOJ/FTC conclude that the joint venture agreement between competitors has not caused and is unlikely to cause anticompetitive harm, the inquiry is at an end and the joint venture can be (or continue to be) effectuated. In the unusual circumstance that DOJ/FTC determine that the joint venture arrangement has caused or is likely to cause anticompetitive harm, the agencies will permit the arrangement only if the potential anticompetitive harm is exceeded by cognizable efficiencies benefiting consumers for which the joint venture is "reasonably necessary."[48] Possible efficiencies include economies of scale, provision of new technologies not otherwise affordable, and combinations of complementary resources or expertise.[49] The agencies will acknowledge a given efficiency only if there are reasonable means to (1) substantiate the likelihood and magnitude of the efficiency, (2) determine how and when the efficiency will be achieved, (3) assess the costs of achieving the efficiency, and (4) project how the efficiency would enhance the venture's and/or participants' ability to compete.[50] Vague and speculative efficiencies will not be acknowledged, nor will cost savings arising from anticompetitive output or service reductions.[51]

Certain categories of arrangements pose such a low risk of anticompetitive effect relative to procompetitive efficiencies that DOJ/FTC has asserted a priori that it will not challenge them except in "extraordinary circumstances." These categories are referred to as antitrust safety zones. The following are the recognized safety zones most pertinent to hospital joint ventures:

- **Joint Ventures Generally:** Agreements that are not *per se* illegal and involve a joint venture arrangement in which the joint venture and its participants collectively maintain a market share of no more than 20% in each relevant market in which competition may be affected.[52]

- **Joint Ventures Involving Expensive Medical Equipment:** Joint ventures in which (1) the joint venture participants are hospitals, (2) the joint venture is limited to the acquisition and operation of hi-tech or other expensive health care equipment, and (3) the joint venture is limited to the minimum number of hospitals necessary to "support the equipment."[53]

Caveats

If the parties to an actual or existing joint venture are uncertain as to whether an actual or proposed joint venture would produce procompetitive efficiencies exceeding potential anticompetitive harm, they can seek a business review letter on the arrangement from DOJ or an advisory opinion regarding the arrangement from the FTC. In doing so, however, parties should be mindful that (1) it will likely take months to secure a response from the government, (2) seeking such a determination might raise the joint venture's profile with federal regulators, and (3) a positive advisory opinion or business review letter will only afford protection on a prospective basis.

It should be noted that the competitive effects of an agreement may change over time due to internal changes within the joint venture or evolving market conditions.[54] DOJ/FTC reserve the right to review arrangements on an ongoing basis and to mandate changes as necessary after the inception of a venture.[55]

Even when a joint venture clearly has a procompetitive effect, DOJ/FTC will examine whether it includes collateral arrangements that are (1) not reasonably necessary to secure the efficiencies sought by the joint venture and (2) unreasonably restrict competition.[56]

Contracting Joint Ventures

Antitrust compliance concerns are not limited to Clinical Joint Ventures. Hospitals must also be cognizant of federal antitrust law when forming and operating a joint venture with area providers in an effort to facilitate contract negotiations with private payors. These joint ventures can take the form of a formal physician–hospital organization or ("PHO") or less formal contractual arrangements between independent providers resulting in a multiprovider network. The antitrust concerns associated with each are similar, and they are therefore addressed collectively herein as "Contracting Joint Ventures."

Antitrust concerns with Contracting Joint Ventures vary substantially depending upon whether the Contracting Joint Venture involves price-fixing arrangements among competing providers.

Contracting Joint Ventures Involving Price Fixing

Government scrutiny will be greatest in connection with the establishment of Contracting Joint Ventures that prospectively fix prices to be charged by providers for the services furnished through the arrangement.[57] The paramount factor in determining the permissibility of such joint ventures is whether they involve actual integration among the participating providers. If such integration is absent, any effort by participating providers to jointly fix prices will likely be condemned as a *per se* violation of federal antitrust law.[58] If, however, there is sufficient integration among the participating providers within the Contracting Joint Venture to achieve efficiencies benefiting consumers, (e.g., quality assurance, reduced administrative costs, economies of scale), and if any agreement relating to price or other matters is "reasonably necessary" to realize those efficiencies, DOJ/FTC will apply a "rule of reason" analysis in assessing its legality.[59]

Integration Among Participating Providers Providers participating in a Contracting Joint Venture can achieve cost efficiencies benefiting consumers (and potentially justifying joint pricing) through financial or clinical integration. Again, the key factors for DOJ/FTC will be whether (1) the degree of integration among participating providers is sufficient to generate cost efficiencies benefiting consumers and (2) any associated agreement among participating providers is sufficiently related to the achievement of these efficiencies.[60]

DOJ/FTC have provided little guidance as to what types of clinical integration might suffice to support a rule-of-reason analysis. Rather, they insist that the diverse array of providers and diverse means of clinical integration inhibit their ability to provide general guidance.[61] As a result, reliance upon clinical integration alone between providers poses some regulatory risk, which is further exacerbated by the greater difficulty in establishing that an associated agreement relating to joint pricing is related to the achievement of clinical integration.

Recently, however, the FTC did provide some of the more significant guidance regarding types of clinical integration that might support a price-fixing arrangement. Specifically, the FTC issued an advisory opinion to MedSouth, Inc., concluding that a nonexclusive independent practice association ("IPA") in which the IPA negotiated fee-for-service rates with third-party payors would not presently warrant a regulatory enforcement action in light of the significant clinical integration fostered by the IPA.[62] Specifically, the IPA proposed to develop and implement the following mechanisms for clinical integration: (1) establishment of a web-based clinical data record utilized by all IPA members to share medical records, access test results, and transfer physician orders; (2) development and adoption of common clinical protocols for specific diagnoses; (3) development and monitoring of physician performance against clinical benchmarks; and (4) termination of physicians who fail to meet specified quality standards. The FTC concluded that the IPA's ability to negotiate common fee-for-service rates through the non-exclusive IPA was reasonably related to the achievement the procompetitive efficiencies associated with integration. In doing so, the FTC emphasized that the IPA would be non-exclusive and further noted that the IPA would retain an independent consultant who would submit bids on its behalf while preventing the disclosure of competitive information among its members.

Most Contracting Joint Ventures rely on financial integration as the basis to support joint pricing strategies. DOJ/FTC recognize that the ability of participating providers to collectively set prices within markets is often an "integral part" of generating the cost efficiencies benefiting consumers, and therefore warrants rule-of-reason analysis.[63] FTC/DOJ have recognized that substantial financial integration within a Contracting Joint Venture can be achieved through the following (as well as other mechanisms):

- Agreement by the Contracting Joint Venture to provide services to a payor at a "capitated rate."

- Agreement by the Contracting Joint Venture to provide designated services or classes of health services to a health plan for a predetermined percent of premium or revenue from the plan.

- Agreement by the Contracting Joint Venture to provide "significant financial incentives" to its participating providers "as a group" to achieve specified cost-containment goals (e.g., substantial withholds from payments to all participating providers with later distribution predicated upon network-wide realization of specified cost-containment goals or substantial rewards or penalties associated with venture-wide achievement of specified cost or utilization targets).

- Agreement by the Contracting Joint Venture to provide a "complex or extended course of treatment" that requires "substantial coordination of care by different types of providers offering complementary services for a fixed, predetermined amount" and for which the cost can vary greatly.[64]

Rule-of-Reason Analysis   Upon concluding that a Contracting Joint Venture involves the requisite level of integration, DOJ/FTC will review any agreement among participating providers relating to joint pricing under a rule-of-reason analysis.[65]

First, DOJ/FTC will analyze the effect of the Contracting Joint Venture on general competition in the geographic area among providers within each of the clinical service lines included in the joint venture (i.e., horizontal competition).[66] This involves a determination as to whether the Contracting Joint Venture would give rise to sufficient market concentration in a given service line (e.g., hospital services) to permit the venture to raise prices charged for that service.[67] One significant factor in determining market concentration and purchaser autonomy is whether the Contracting Joint Venture is "exclusive" (i.e., whether network providers are required to furnish their services exclusively through the network).[68] Although exclusive Contracting Joint Venture arrangements are not impermissible *per se*, they raise heightened antitrust concerns given that providers are not free to compete on the basis of price outside the joint venture framework.[69] If a Contracting Joint Venture is exclusive, the government will assess the market share of the providers in each clinical service line who are subject to the exclusivity requirement, duration of the exclusivity period, the providers' ability to withdraw from the network arrangement, the financial incentives or disincentives relating to withdrawal, the number of providers that must be included in the joint venture for it to compete effectively, and the purported justification for the exclusivity arrangement.[70] Another key consideration is whether health plans and other purchasers are willing and able to switch networks within a market in response to a price increase imposed by the Contracting Joint Venture.[71]

Second, DOJ/FTC will analyze the effect of the Contracting Joint Venture on competition in the geographic area with other Contracting Joint Ventures (i.e., vertical competition).[72] Specifically, the government will scrutinize whether the joint venture arrangement involves commitments from constituent providers that would preclude the ability of other Contracting Joint Ventures or noncontracting health plans to compete in the market.[73] The principal concern will be whether a given Contracting Joint Venture has exclusive arrangements with a large percentage of a given type of physician (e.g., obstetricians) or specialized provider (e.g., skilled nursing facilities) to prevent other purchasers, payors, or providers from forming an alternative network.[74] In making this assessment, the government will review the same aspects of the exclusivity agreements as it does in assessing horizontal competition.[75]

Finally, if a Contracting Joint Venture gives rise to horizontal or vertical competitiveness concerns, DOJ/FTC will assess whether it will directly result in countervailing efficiencies that (1) will outweigh any potential anticompetitive effects and result in lower costs or higher quality and (2) cannot be achieved through less anticompetitive means.[76] In general DOJ/FTC believe that the extent of efficiencies generated through a Contracting Joint Venture (e.g., cost controls, quality assurance, economies of scale, reduced administrative costs) will correlate with the degree of financial and clinical integration.[77] Moreover, DOJ/FTC assert that the more competition facing the joint venture, the greater the likely cost reductions and quality improvements to be produced through such integration.[78]

Contracting Joint Ventures Not Involving Price Fixing

Contracting Joint Ventures that do not involve joint pricing among participating providers pose little risk under federal antitrust laws. The most common form of such a network arrangement is the so-called messenger model PHO.[79] Under this arrangement, the participating providers use the Contracting Joint Venture as an independent agent to convey to purchasers the price-related terms the individual provider is willing to accept.[80] Providers in such a Contracting Joint Venture typically do not integrate, financially or clinically, in any meaningful way.[81] DOJ/FTC believe such arrangements raise little concern under federal antitrust law so long as they neither create nor facilitate a collective agreement among participating providers on price or price-related terms.[82] The government will heavily scrutinize such arrangements to ensure that this condition is met. These unintegrated Contracting Joint Ventures will likely be deemed to violate federal antitrust law if they move beyond the role of conduit between individual providers and purchasers and attempt to (1) disseminate the views or intentions of a participating provider regarding a proposal from/to a purchaser, (2) express opinion on the terms offered by or to be offered to a purchaser, or (3) exercise independent judgment as to whether a given offer is sufficiently attractive to be conveyed to or from a provider.[83]

Disclosure of Information Between Competitors in Connection with a Joint Venture

Establishment and ongoing operation of a Clinical or Administrative joint venture can result in the disclosure of information between actual or potential competitors. Such disclosure could arise when competitors engaged in a joint venture exchange information on topics not reasonably necessary for efficient operation of the venture or when the joint venture itself exchanges information with an actual or potential competitor. Disclosure in either context can raise antitrust concerns. Specifically, DOJ/FTC will inquire whether the information disclosed could serve as a basis for competitors to collude in setting prices and compensation terms within their market.[84] The appropriate analysis and pertinent safeguards will vary slightly depending upon the type of information involved.

Price- or Compensation-Related Information

Disclosures among competitors of current or future pricing or current or future personnel compensation levels will "very likely" be considered anti-competitive by DOJ/FTC.[85] Competitors considering such activity could consider securing an advisory opinion from the FTC or a business review letter from DOJ. Competitors should note that if the disclosures result in agreement among them as to prices or compensation, the arrangement will likely be deemed unlawful *per se*.[86]

DOJ/FTC do, however, grant actual or potential competitors substantially more leeway to disclose fee-related information in connection with (1) a third-party survey of prices and compensation within a given industry or (2) a collective submission of fee information to (and at the request of) purchasers of health care services. Indeed, DOJ/FTC recognize that, while such disclosures do pose some risk of facilitating anticompetitive collusion, they can also have pro-competitive benefits by permitting purchasers and consumers to make more informed decisions in choosing their provider, permitting providers to price their services more competitively, and permitting providers to offer competitive salaries and benefits to attract workers.[87]

Consequently, DOJ/FTC have developed an "antitrust safety zone" to protect participation in surveys or collective submissions involving fee-related information, submissions that are likely to promote competition and provide minimal basis for anticompetitive collusion.[88] Participation in a survey in accord with safety zone requirements will not result in antitrust liability "absent extraordinary circumstances."[89] Safety zone protection will be afforded when each of the following requirements is met: (1) the survey/information collection is managed by an independent third-party (e.g., purchaser, government agency, health care consultant, trade association, and so on), (2) the information provided by competing participants is based on data more than three months old, (3) each published survey statistic or disclosure is based upon data from at least five providers, (4) no individual provider's data represents more than 25% of the weighted basis of any published survey statistic or disclosure, and (5) information published in the survey or disclosures is sufficiently aggregated that one cannot identify the prices charged or compensation paid by any individual participant.[90] It should be noted that the antitrust safety zone does not protect attempts by competitors to use the survey information or disclosures as a basis to collusively insist on specified terms from purchasers or to threaten to boycott those purchasers refusing to meet certain demands to collectively refuse to negotiate with purchasers. Indeed, such activity would likely constitute a *per se* violation of federal antitrust laws.[91]

Disclosures among competitors outside the antitrust safety zone will be reviewed by DOJ/FTC on a case-by-case basis. DOJ/FTC will assess whether the procompetitive effects of the disclosures at issue outweigh the risk that they could serve as a basis for collusion among competitors vis-à-vis purchasers.[92] The risk of collusion will likely be reduced when the survey or collective disclosure is managed by a third party that aggregates information before dissemination among competitors, the information disclosed by the providers is historical in nature, or there is a broad array of competitors contributing information in connection with the survey.[93] If competing providers are concerned that participation in a survey or other collective disclosure of information might raise significant antitrust concerns, they could consider seeking an advisory opinion from the FTC and/or a business review letter from DOJ.

Information Relating to Matters Other Than Price and Compensation

DOJ/FTC conclude that the exchange of information among competitors on matters other than price and compensation poses less risk of anticompetitive collusion when the exchange is undertaken for the purpose of making a collective disclosure for consideration by a purchaser.[94] DOJ/FTC have specifically created an "antitrust safety zone" to protect the collection and sharing of medical outcome data as well as the use of such data in developing suggested clinical practice parameters for treating various clinical indications.[95] Competing providers are, however, strictly prohibited from collectively threatening to boycott a purchaser who refuses to adhere to the foregoing clinical parameters.[96] Indeed, providers who collectively threaten to deal with a purchaser because they object to the purchaser's administrative, clinical, or other terms run a "substantial risk" under the federal antitrust laws.[97]

Disclosures of information among competitors on other matters outside the realm of price and compensation terms will not enjoy the protection of an antitrust safety zone, but generally pose less risk of anticompetitive collusion and, therefore, are less likely to be challenged.[98] Nonetheless, if the nature of the information to be exchanged could reasonably be deemed to serve as the basis for anticompetitive collusion among competitors, the parties could seek an advisory opinion from the FTC or a business review letter from DOJ in advance of such disclosures.

ENDNOTES

1. Many states have adopted antitrust restrictions that may be implicated by a joint venture arrangement. Although such laws are beyond the scope of this work, special care must be taken to ensure compliance with these state restrictions.

2. 15 U.S.C. § 1. "Although the Sherman Act, by its terms, prohibits every agreement 'in restraint of trade,'" the Supreme Court "has long recognized that Congress intended to outlaw only unreasonable restraints." *State Oil Co. v. Kahn*, 522 U.S. 3, 10 (1997).

3. 15 U.S.C. § 2.

4. 15 U.S.C. §§ 1, 2; 18 U.S.C. § 3571.

5. 15 U.S.C. §§ 1, 2; 18 U.S.C. § 3571.

6. 15 U.S.C. § 1322 et. seq.

7. 15 U.S.C. § 18. The mere acquisition of equity for investment purposes will not implicate the Clayton Act. 15 U.S.C. § 18.

8. 15 U.S.C. §§ 45, 53, 1311–1314.

9. 15 U.S.C. §§ 15(a), 15a.

10. 15 U.S.C. § 45. See, for example, *FTC v. Brown Shoe Co.*, 384 U.S. 316, 322 (1966) (defining "unfair trade practices" under 15 U.S.C. § 45 to include violations of the Sherman and Clayton acts) (citation and ellipses omitted).

11. 15 U.S.C. § 45.

12. *Cal. Dental Assn v. FTC*, 526 U.S. 756, 765-769 (1999).

13. 15 U.S.C. §§ 4301-4306.

14. 15 U.S.C. § 4302.

15. 15 U.S.C. § 4301(b).

16. 15 U.S.C. § 4303.

17. 15 U.S.C. § 18a; 42 C.F.R. § 801.90(b)-(c).

18. See, for example, FTC Premerger Notification Office, Formal Interpretation 15 (March 2001) Formal Interpretation 15 at 4.

19. See, for example, Formal Interpretation 15 at 4. Note that the contribution of intellectual property to a joint venture is deemed the contribution of a business for purposes of triggering the HSR requirement. Formal Interpretation 15 at 4–5.

20. 16 C.F.R. § 801.40(c).

21. *City of Columbia v. Omni Outdoor Advertising*, 499 U.S. 365, 370 (1991).

22. DOJ/FTC Health Industry Guidelines §§ 1.2, 2.1, 3.1; DOJ/FTC Collaboration Guidelines §§ 2.1, 3.31(a).

23. DOJ/FTC Collaboration Guidelines § 1.1 n.6.

24. DOJ/FTC Health Industry Guidelines §§ 1.2, 2.1, 3.1; DOJ/FTC Collaboration Guidelines §§ 2.2, 3.31(a), 3.31(b); DOJ/FTC Merger Guidelines § 0.1.

25. DOJ/FTC Collaboration Guidelines §§ 2.2, 3.1(a) n. 37, 3.31(b).

26. DOJ/FTC Collaboration Guidelines §§ 1.2, 2.1, 3.1, 3.3.

27. DOJ/FTC Collaboration Guidelines §§ 1.2, 2.1, 3.1, 3.3. Application of this standard is mandated by statute in connection with joint ventures for the provision of items and services as well as joint ventures for certain research activities. 15 U.S.C. § 4302.

28. DOJ/FTC Collaboration Guidelines § 3.32(a); DOJ/FTC Merger Guidelines § 1.0, referenced in DOJ/FTC Collaboration Guidelines § 3.32(a).

29. DOJ/FTC Collaboration Guidelines § 3.32(a); DOJ/FTC Merger Guidelines § 1.11, referenced in DOJ/FTC Collaboration Guidelines § 3.32(a).

30. DOJ/FTC Merger Guidelines § 1.21, referenced in DOJ/FTC Collaboration Guidelines § 3.32(a).

31. DOJ/FTC Collaboration Guidelines § 3.33.

32. DOJ/FTC Collaboration Guidelines § 3.33.

33. DOJ/FTC Merger Guidelines § 2.2, referenced in DOJ/FTC Collaboration Guidelines § 3.33.

34. DOJ/FTC Merger Guidelines § 2.2, referenced in DOJ/FTC Collaboration Guidelines § 3.33.

35. DOJ/FTC Merger Guidelines § 2.2, referenced in DOJ/FTC Collaboration Guidelines § 3.33.

36. DOJ/FTC Merger Guidelines § 2.2, referenced in DOJ/FTC Collaboration Guidelines § 3.33.

37. DOJ/FTC Merger Guidelines §§ 2.1, 2.11, referenced in DOJ/FTC Collaboration Guidelines § 3.33.

38. DOJ/FTC Merger Guidelines § 2.1, referenced in DOJ/FTC Collaboration Guidelines § 3.33. DOJ/FTC will recognize that market share and market concentration may overstate one's market power if one can identify ongoing market changes (e.g., technological developments) that might make historical market share and market concentration a less effective proxy for likely future trends. DOJ/FTC Merger Guidelines 1.52, referenced in, DOJ/FTC Collaboration Guidelines § 3.33.

39. DOJ/FTC Collaboration Guidelines § 3.35.

40. DOJ/FTC Collaboration Guidelines § 3.35.

41. DOJ/FTC Collaboration Guidelines § 3.34.

42. DOJ/FTC Collaboration Guidelines § 3.34(a).

43. DOJ/FTC Collaboration Guidelines § 3.34(f).

44. DOJ/FTC Collaboration Guidelines § 3.34(b).

45. DOJ/FTC Collaboration Guidelines § 3.34(c).

46. DOJ/FTC Collaboration Guidelines § 3.34(d).

47. DOJ/FTC Collaboration Guidelines § 3.34(e).

48. DOJ/FTC Collaboration Guidelines §§ 3.36, 3.37.

49. DOJ/FTC Health Industry Guidelines §§ 2, 3; DOJ/FTC Collaboration Guidelines §§ 2.1, 3.31(a).

50. DOJ/FTC Collaboration Guidelines § 3.36(a).

51. DOJ/FTC Collaboration Guidelines § 3.36(b).

52. DOJ/FTC Collaboration Guidelines § 4.2.

53. DOJ/FTC Health Industry Guidelines §§ 2(A), 3(A). In determining the number of hospitals needed to support the pertinent equipment, DOJ and the FTC will determine (1) the cost of the equipment, (2) the equipment's remaining useful life, (3) the expected payment for each procedure, (4) the number of procedures needed to break even, and (5) the likely number of procedures annually from each hospital given its service area. DOJ/FTC Health Industry Guidelines §§ 2(A), 3(A).

54. DOJ/FTC Collaboration Guidelines § 2.4.

55. DOJ/FTC Collaboration Guidelines § 2.4.

56. DOJ/FTC Health Industry Guidelines §§ 2(B), 3(B).

57. DOJ/FTC Health Industry Guidelines § 9.

58. DOJ/FTC Health Industry Guidelines § 9.

59. DOJ/FTC Health Industry Guidelines § 9.

60. DOJ/FTC Health Industry Guidelines § 9(A).

61. DOJ/FTC Health Industry Guidelines § 9(A).

62. FTC Advisory Opinion regarding MedSouth, Inc. (Feb. 19, 2002).

63. DOJ/FTC Health Industry Guidelines § 9(A).

64. DOJ/FTC Health Industry Guidelines § 9(A).

65. DOJ/FTC Health Industry Guidelines § 9(B)(1)-(2).

66. DOJ/FTC Health Industry Guidelines § 9(B)(2)(a).

67. DOJ/FTC Health Industry Guidelines § 9(B)(2)(a).

68. DOJ/FTC Health Industry Guidelines § 9(B)(2)(a). DOJ/FTC will look behind the terms of the network agreement in making this inquiry. Thus, if network providers are exclusively (or almost exclusively) furnishing their services through the network, the network will be deemed exclusive even if exclusivity is disclaimed in the network affiliation agreement. DOJ Health Industry Guidelines § 9(B)(2)(a). Moreover, DOJ/FTC will apply the same scrutiny when reviewing restrictions on the ability of a network provider to furnish services outside of the network, even when such restrictions fall short of outright exclusivity. DOJ/FTC Health Industry Guidelines § 9(B)(2)(a).

69. DOJ/FTC Health Industry Guidelines § 9(B)(2)(a).

70. DOJ/FTC Health Industry Guidelines § 9(B)(2)(a).

71. DOJ/FTC Health Industry Guidelines § 9(B)(2)(a).

72. DOJ/FTC Health Industry Guidelines § 9(B)(2)(b).

73. DOJ/FTC Health Industry Guidelines § 9(B)(2)(b).

74. DOJ/FTC Health Industry Guidelines § 9(B)(2)(b).

75. DOJ/FTC Health Industry Guidelines § 9(B)(2)(b).

76. DOJ/FTC Health Industry Guidelines § 9(B)(3).

77. DOJ/FTC Health Industry Guidelines § 9(B)(3).

78. DOJ/FTC Health Industry Guidelines § 9(B)(3).

79. DOJ/FTC Health Industry Guidelines § 9(C).

80. DOJ/FTC Health Industry Guidelines § 9(C).

81. DOJ/FTC Health Industry Guidelines § 9(C).

82. DOJ/FTC Health Industry Guidelines § 9(C).

83. DOJ/FTC Health Industry Guidelines § 9(C).

84. DOJ/FTC Health Industry Guidelines §§ 4-6.

85. DOJ/FTC Health Industry Guidelines §§ 5(B), 6(B).

86. DOJ/FTC Health Industry Guidelines §§ 5(B), 6(B).

87. DOJ/FTC Health Industry Guidelines §§ 5, 6.

88. DOJ/FTC Health Industry Guidelines §§ 5(A), 6(A).

89. DOJ/FTC Health Industry Guidelines §§ 5(A), 6(A).

90. DOJ/FTC Health Industry Guidelines §§ 5(A), 6(A).

91. DOJ/FTC Health Industry Guidelines §§ 5(B), 6(B).

92. DOJ/FTC Health Industry Guidelines §§ 5(B), 6(B).

93. DOJ/FTC Health Industry Guidelines §§ 5(B), 6(B).

94. DOJ/FTC Health Industry Guidelines § 4.

95. DOJ/FTC Health Industry Guidelines § 4(A).

96. DOJ/FTC Health Industry Guidelines § 4(A).

97. DOJ/FTC Health Industry Guidelines § 4(A).

98. DOJ/FTC Health Industry Guidelines § 4.

CHAPTER 5

Federal Securities Laws Affecting Hospital Joint Ventures

INTRODUCTION

When raising capital through the issuance of equity or debt, joint venture representatives must take special care to ensure compliance with federal securities laws. Failure to do so can result in liability on the part of the joint venture as well as those promoting the joint venture's securities.[1]

OVERVIEW OF FEDERAL SECURITIES LAWS

The Securities Act of 1933 ("Securities Act") generally requires that an entity planning to offer or sell securities register them in advance with the Securities and Exchange Commission ("SEC"). Violation of the registration requirements of the Securities Act may subject an issuer and any individuals deemed to be promoters, to civil and criminal penalties from the SEC and to liability for rescission of the purchase price to any individual purchasing the unregistered security.[2] The registration process, however, is both expensive and time consuming. Additionally, registration may subject the joint venture to ongoing reporting and other requirements under the Securities Act and Securities and Exchange Act of 1934 ("Exchange Act"). Thus, joint venture representatives will most often structure their securities offerings so as to qualify for an exemption from the Securities Act registration requirements.[3]

APPLICATION TO HOSPITAL JOINT VENTURES

Determining Whether a Financial Instrument Is A "Security"

Although the Securities Act is only implicated if a joint venture offers or sells an instrument that qualifies as a "security," the term is applied with sufficient breadth by the SEC and federal courts that the venture should assume that any corporate stock, limited partnership interest, or limited liability company membership interest would be considered a security under the Act.[4] Promissory notes issued by a joint venture will also presumptively be deemed securities for purposes of the Securities Act.[5] Exceptions may apply for (1) notes executed in connection with a traditional commercial loan, (2) notes executed as part of an "open-account relationship" with a lending institution, and (3) short-term commercial paper.[6]

Exemption from Registration Requirements of the Securities Act

There are a variety of bases upon which to exempt joint venture securities from the registration requirement of the Securities Act. The principal bases are described below.

Intrastate Offerings

Overview When a joint venture will furnish services exclusively in the state in which it is organized and in which all investors reside, the joint venture may wish to rely on the nonexclusive exemption for intrastate offerings as the principal basis for exemption from the registration requirements of the Securities Act. Reliance on this exemption affords numerous benefits.

First, so long as the joint venture's patient base and investors reside in a single state, the exemption poses few constraints on the activities that the joint venture would otherwise undertake. Second, the joint venture will not be obligated to make the often difficult determination, required for compliance with other exemptions under the Securities Act, as to whether a potential investor may properly be deemed an Accredited Investor or a Qualified Investor. Third, the exemption is less restrictive than other exemptions with respect to the method and manner in which the offering is advertised. Fourth, if an exemption requirement is inadvertently violated, the joint venture might have a credible argument that the statutory exception for intrastate offerings under the Securities Act is broader than the exemption (i.e., the exemption is nonexclusive), and violation of the exemption does not preclude statutory protection. Finally, if the size of an offering is sufficiently small and solicitation is made discreetly, the joint venture could argue that it is further protected by the statutory exception for private offerings described later in this chapter in the section entitled Private Placement Exception.

Statutory Exception Section 3(a)(11) of the Securities Act provides that the registration provisions of the Securities Act do not apply to securities that are sold by the issuer only in a single state in which it is doing business (and, if a corporation, the state in which it is incorporated and doing business) and sold only to those residing in that state.[7]

Nonexclusive Exemption The SEC has promulgated Rule 147 as an exemption to assist issuers relying on the § 3(a)(11). Transactions complying with the exemption are assured of protection under § 3(a)(11), while transactions outside the exempt may or may not enjoy such protection.[8] In order to secure exempt status, all offers and sales made in connection with an issue of securities must comport with the exemption.[9] In order to qualify, the issuer must make all offers and sales to residents of the state in which the issuer is "resident and doing business." [10] An issuer is deemed to "reside" in the jurisdiction in which it is organized or incorporated. An issuer is deemed to be "doing business" within the state if all of the following hold true:

- Eighty percent of its gross revenues came from rendering services in the state or the operation of a business or ownership of realty in the state.

- In the most recent semiannual fiscal period prior to the first offer in the issue, 80% of the issuer's assets were located in the jurisdiction.

- The issuer uses 80% of the net proceeds it receives from the issue in connection with the operation of a business, purchase of realty, or furnishing of services within such state or territory.

- The state is the issuer's principal place of business.[11]

For nine months after the last sale in the given issue, all resales must be made only to persons resident in the state in which the offering occurred.[12] The issuer must take a number of steps to prevent interstate resales. First, the issuer must place a legend on the securities indicating that they have not been registered under the Securities Act and cannot be sold outside the state for nine months after the last sale involving the issue.[13] Second, the issuer must issue stop transfer instructions during the nine-month period.[14] Third, the issuer must obtain a written representation from each purchaser as to the purchaser's residence.[15] The issuer must provide written disclosure of the restrictions on, and the foregoing safeguards against, resale.[16]

Regulation D

If a joint venture cannot be certain that it will furnish services exclusively in the jurisdiction in which it is organized, or if it cannot raise sufficient capital from residents of that jurisdiction, it might choose to rely on one of the exemptions codified in Regulation D. Regulation D comprises three distinct exemptions from the registration requirements of the Securities Act.[17] These exemptions concern offerings not exceeding $1 million, those not exceeding $5 million, and offerings exceeding $5 million.

Offering Not Exceeding $1 Million. Nonpublicly traded entities conducting an offering that will not exceed $1 million may qualify under Rule 504 for exemption from the registration requirements associated with the Securities Act.[18] There is no ceiling on the number of purchasers who may participate in the issue. Unlike the other Regulation D exemptions, there are no mandated disclosures to investors prior to sale or limits on the number of offerees.

Requirements Relating to the Manner of Solicitation

An issuer relying on Rule 504 may not offer the securities through a "general solicitation" or "general advertising" (which includes solicitations or advertisements through periodicals, through the broadcast media, or at seminars or meetings advertised through periodicals or the broadcast media).[19] Generally, compliance with the general solicitation requirement permits offers only to persons previously known to the solicitor. Exception is made, however, in two circumstances. First, the restriction on general solicitation will not apply with respect to an issuer that offers and sells securities exclusively in a state in which the issuer (1) is required by state law to file a written disclosure statement with the state regarding the issue, (2) is required by state law to furnish such disclosure statement to investors prior to the sale of any securities from the issue, and (3) complies with these requirements.[20]

Second, the restriction will not apply with respect to an issue made in accordance with state law disclosure exemptions that permit general solicitation and advertising regarding the issue so long as sales are made only to accredited investors ("Accredited Investors").[21] Accredited Investors include, under certain circumstances, the following:

- Banks.

- Securities brokers and dealers registered with the SEC.

- Insurance companies.

- Investment companies registered with the SEC.

- Employee benefit plans.

- State benefit plans.

- Exempt organizations, partnerships, corporations, and business trusts maintaining over $5,000,000 in assets and not formed for purposes of acquiring the securities at issue.

- Directors, executive officers, or general partners of the issuer.

- Directors, executive officers, or general partners of a general partner of the issuer.

- Natural persons whose household net worth exceeds $1,000,000.

- Natural persons whose individual income exceeds $200,000 in each of the two most recent years and is reasonably expected to reach the same income level in the current year.

- Natural persons whose joint household income exceeds $300,000 in each of the two most recent years and is reasonably expected to reach the same income level in the current year.

- A trust with assets in excess of $5 million that was not formed for the specific purpose of acquiring the securities offered and that is directed by a "sophisticated person."

- An entity in which all equity owners are accredited investors.[22]

Requirements Relating to Resale

An issuer relying on this exemption must also take reasonable care to ensure that those purchasing securities are doing so for investment purposes and not with the intent to resell them.[23] The SEC has recognized that one method of exercising reasonable care is to (1) "make reasonable inquiry to determine the purchaser is acquiring the securities for himself or other persons," (2) make written disclosure to each purchaser prior to sale that the securities have not been registered under the Securities Act and cannot be resold absent registration or an applicable exemption from the registration requirement, and (3) placement of a legend on the document constituting the security that references restrictions on the transferability and sale of the securities.[24]

As with the requirements relating to the manner of investor solicitation, the requirements relating to resale are inapplicable under either of two circumstances. First, the restriction will not apply with respect to an issuer that (1) is required by state law to file a written disclosure statement with the state regarding the issue, (2) is required by state law to furnish such disclosure statement to investors prior to the sale of any securities from the issue, and (3) complies with these requirements.[25] Second, the restriction will not apply with respect to an issue made in accordance with state law disclosure exemptions that permit general solicitation and advertising regarding the issue so long as sales are made only to accredited investors.[26]

Offering Not Exceeding $5 Million. An entity contemplating an offering that will not exceed $5 million may qualify under Rule 505 for exemption from the registration requirements associated with the Securities Act.[27] Entities that directly or through their predecessors or affiliates, are party to (or have been sanctioned in) certain administrative or judicial proceedings relating to federal securities laws are precluded from relying upon this exception.[28]

Requirements Regarding the Number of Purchasers

The issuer must reasonably believe that there are no more than 35 purchasers in the offering.[29] The number of purchasers shall not include:

- Accredited Investors.[30]

- Any relative of the purchaser (by blood or marriage) living at another purchaser's principal residence ("Qualified Relative"). [31]

- Any trust or estate in which a purchaser or any of his or her Qualified Relatives collectively own more than 50% beneficial interest.[32]

- Any organization of which a purchaser and any of his or her Qualified Relatives are beneficial owners of more than 50% of the equity securities.

Requirements Regarding the Manner of Solicitation

An issuer relying on this exception may not offer the securities through a "general solicitation" or "general advertising" (e.g., solicitations or advertisements through periodicals, through the broadcast media, or at seminars or meetings advertised through periodicals or the broadcast media).[33] As with Rule 504 offerings, offerees must generally be known to the solicitors.

Requirements Regarding Disclosures

Prior to selling a security to an investor, other than an Accredited Investor, the issuer must furnish certain written materials.[34] The requisite type and scope of disclosures vary depending upon the size of the issue and type of entity issuing securities and may include audited or unaudited financial statements as well as other information.[35] Material information provided to Accredited Investors in connection with the issue must be briefly described to nonaccredited investors and made available to them upon request prior to the sale.[36] Prior to the sale, the issuer must also make available to each Nonaccredited Investor the "opportunity to ask question and receive answers concerning the terms and conditions of the offering and obtain any additional information which the issuer possesses or can acquire without unreasonable effort or expense that is necessary to verify the accuracy of the information" included in the mandatory written disclosures.[37] Written disclosure must also be provided to Nonaccredited Investors regarding the restriction on resale of the securities.[38]

Requirements Regarding Resale

An issuer relying on Rule 505 must take reasonable care to ensure that those purchasing securities are doing so for investment purposes and not with the intent to resell them.[39] The SEC has recognized that one method of exercising reasonable care is to (1) make reasonable inquiry to determine the purchaser is acquiring the securities for himself or other persons, (2) make written disclosure to each purchaser prior to sale that the securities have not been registered under the Securities Act and cannot be resold absent registration or an applicable exemption from the registration requirement, and (3) placement of a legend on the document constituting the security, which references restrictions on the transferability and sale of the securities.[40]

Offering Exceeding $5 Million An entity contemplating an offering that will exceed $5 million may qualify under Rule 506 for exemption from the registration requirements associated with the Securities Act. The Rule 506 requirements are identical to those of Rule 505 for an offering not exceeding $5 million, with only two exceptions. First, there is no limitation on the size of the issue.[41] Second, Nonaccredited investors must meet certain qualifications. Specifically, the issuer must reasonably conclude at the time of purchase that each of the Nonaccredited Investors has "such knowledge and experience in financial and business matters that he is capable of evaluating the merits and risks of the prospective investment" ("Qualified Investor").[42] In assessing whether a potential investor is a Qualified Investor, the issuer may—under certain circumstances—impute to the investor the knowledge of investor representatives relied upon by the purchaser if such representatives have no conflict of interest and "have such knowledge and experience in financial and business matters that [they] are capable of evaluating . . . the merits and risks of the prospective investment" to the purchaser.[43] Thus, an individual who would not otherwise qualify as a Qualified Investor may be deemed such when the issuer knows he or she is using a Qualified Purchaser or Representative.[44]

Accredited Investors Exception

Section 4(6) of the Securities Act provides that the disclosure provisions of the Act do not apply to the placement of an issue if (1) offers or sales are made solely to "accredited investors," (2) the aggregate offering price of the issue does not exceed $5 million, and (3) there is no "advertising or public solicitation" in connection with the issue.[45] The term accredited investor has a similar meaning as in Regulation D.[46]

Private Placement Exception

Section 4(2) of the Securities Act provides that the registration requirements of the Securities Act do not apply to a transaction not involving a public offering of securities.[47] There is no specificity, however, as to precisely what constitutes such an offering. Therefore, issuers typically attempt to comply with Regulation D (described above) so as to be assured of compliance with the Securities Act and use § 4(2) as a fallback. The SEC explicitly states that "an issuer's failure to satisfy all terms and conditions of" Regulation D "shall not raise any presumption that the exemption provided by Section 4(2) of the Act is not available." [48]

Regulation A

In the event that neither the intrastate offering exemption nor the Regulation D exemption is available, Regulation A may afford an exemption from the registration requirements of the Securities Act.[49] Regulation A is generally used as a last resort because it involves a number of restrictions and the filing of an offering statement.

Restrictions on Offer Size The aggregate offering price for the issue cannot exceed $5 million (including no more than $1.5 million offered by all selling security holders).[50] Any sale of securities by the issuer under Regulation A within a twelve-month period must be applied towards this limit.[51]

Restrictions on Making Offers Securities may not be offered for sale until an abbreviated offering statement (including a preliminary offering circular) has been filed with the SEC, though the issuer may conduct certain limited activities "to determine whether there is any interest in a contemplated securities offering." [52] Once such a filing is made, the issuer may (1) conduct certain limited public advertising, (2) make oral offers, and (3) make certain written offers through use of a qualified preliminary offering circular.[53] Once the filing is qualified by the SEC, the issuer may also (1) make other written offers so long as they are accompanied by the approved final offering circular, (2) sell the securities so long as the purchaser receives a preliminary or final offering circular at least 48 hours prior to the confirmation of sale to that person.[54]

Unless an affiliate of the issuer cannot resell the securities in the offering, the issuer has had net income from continuing operations in at least one of the two preceding fiscal years.[55]

Registration, Reporting, and Proxy Requirements of the Securities Act and Exchange Act

In the absence of a public offering, the registration, reporting, and proxy solicitation requirements of the Exchange Act will not apply so long as (1) the issuer's securities are not listed on a national securities exchange and (2) no class of securities is held by 500 or more persons of record.[56] Thus, the central compliance concern remains exemption from the Securities Act, not satisfaction of the reporting and proxy requirements of the Exchange Act.

ENDNOTES

1. Joint venture representatives should note that state securities laws impose additional restrictions governing the issuance, marketing, and sale of securities that supplement, and may be more restrictive than, their federal counterparts. Although such laws are beyond the scope of this work, special care must be taken to ensure compliance with these state restrictions.

2. 15 U.S.C. § 17l(a).

3. Those issuing securities that qualify for exemption from the registration requirement of the Securities Act may still be held liable for civil penalties, criminal penalties, cease and desist orders, injunctions, and civil damages under the antifraud provisions of the Securities Act and the Exchange Act.

4. Corporate stock is almost invariably deemed to be a security. See *Landreth Timber Co. v. Landreth*, 471 U.S. 681, 692 (1985). So are limited partnership interests. *L&B Hosp. Ventures,*

Inc. v. Healthcare Int'l, 894 F.2d 150, 151 (5th Cir. 1990); Carter G. Bishop & Daniel S. Klein-berger, *Limited Liability Companies: Tax and Business Law* (2002) ("Limited Liability Companies") § 11.03[1][c] n.106 (citing cases in which limited partnerships are deemed to be securities for purposes of the Securities Act). Although there are credible grounds to contend that LLC membership interests should rarely qualify as a security, the law is sufficiently ambiguous that a joint venture must assume that such interests would be deemed a security. Limited Liability Companies § 11.03[1]. Finally, although general partnership interests are deemed to be exempt from the definition of a security in many contexts, prudence suggests that it must be assumed that such interests might be deemed security interests in a joint venture context. *Williamson v. Tucker*, 645 F.2d 404, 424 (5th Cir. 1981).

5. *Reves v. Ernst & Young*, 494 U.S. 56, 65 (1990).

6. *Reves*, 494 U.S. at 65, 70-71; 15 U.S.C. §§ 77c(a)(3), 78c(3)(a)(10). Commercial paper is typ-ically deemed to be a negotiable note with a maturity date of less than nine months, which is used to fund ongoing operating expenses and is not made available primarily to the gen-eral public. Zolman Cavitch, *Business Organizations with Tax Planning*, § 93.03[4] (Mathew Bender 2001). The courts and the SEC also make exception for debt notes struc-tured and distributed in such a way that suggests they need not be regulated in order to protect the investing public. *Reves*, 494 U.S. at 65, 70–71; 15 U.S.C. §§ 77c(a)(3), 78c(3)(a)(10). This exception involves application of a number of amorphous factors, however, and therefore should not be relied upon as a prudent basis for negating registra-tion under the Securities Act. See *Reves*, 494 U.S. at 66–67.

7. 16 U.S.C. § 77(c)(11). Section 3(a)(11) and the associated exemption protect an issue of securities from the registration requirements of §§ 5 and 3(a)(11) of the Securities Act but do not afford protection from the antifraud, civil liability, or other provisions in the Act. 17 C.F.R. § 230.147, Preliminary Note 3.

8. 17 C.F.R. § 230.147, Preliminary Note 1.

9. 17 C.F.R. § 230.147(b)(1). An offer or sale of securities by an issuer shall not be deemed to be part of the same issue as a security if at least six months has passed since the last offer, offer for sale, or sale of the same or similar securities by or for the issuer. 17 C.F.R. § 230.147(b)(2). If the issuer has made an offer or sale in connection with a security within the preceding six months, the SEC will assess the following factors in determining whether the previous offer or sale is "part of the same issue": (1) Were the offerings part of the same plan of financing, (2) do the offerings involve issuance of the same class of securities, (3) are the offerings made at or about the same time, (4) is the same type of consideration to be received, and (5) are the offerings made for the same general pur-pose? 17 C.F.R. § 230.147, Preliminary Note 3.

10. 17 C.F.R. § 230.147(c).

11. 17 C.F.R. § 230.147(c)(2). The exemption prescribes various timelines to which these cal-culations apply. 17 C.F.R. § 230.147(c)(2).

12. 17 C.F.R. § 230.147(e).

13. 17 C.F.R. § 230.147(f)(1).

14. 17 C.F.R. § 230.147(f)(1).

15. 17 C.F.R. § 230.147(f)(1).

16. 17 C.F.R. § 230.147(f)(2)-(3).

17. Compliance with any of the three exemptions permits the joint venture to avoid the registration requirements of the Securities Act but does not preclude application of the antifraud, civil liability, or other provisions of federal securities laws. 17 C.F.R. Part 230, Subpart 5, Preliminary Note 1.

18. 17 C.F.R. § 230.504(a). The $1 million threshold includes (1) the securities involved in the issue and (2) all other securities sold by the joint venture during the 12 months preceding conclusion of the offering at issue. 17 C.F.R. § 230.504(b)(2).

19. This restriction also applies to anyone acting on the issuer's behalf.

20. 17 C.F.R. § 230.504(b)(1). If offers and sales are made in multiple jurisdictions and some subset of the jurisdictions does not require the delivery of the substantive disclosure document, the issuer must nonetheless furnish those solicited in such jurisdictions with a copy of the disclosure document prior to sale. 17 C.F.R. § 230.504(b)(1)(ii).

21. 17 C.F.R. § 230.504(b)(1)(iii).

22. 15 U.S.C. § 77b(a)(15); 17 C.F.R. § 230.501(a).

23. 17 C.F.R. § 230.502(d).

24. 17 C.F.R. § 230.503(d). The SEC recognizes that there may be other methods by which to exercise reasonable care to ensure any transfer or resale of the securities comports with the requirements of or exception to the Securities Act. 17 C.F.R. § 230.503(d).

25. 17 C.F.R. § 230.504(b)(1). If offers and sales are made in multiple jurisdictions and some subset of the jurisdictions does not require the delivery of the substantive disclosure document, the issuer must nonetheless furnish those solicited in such jurisdictions with a copy of the disclosure document prior to sale. 17 C.F.R. § 230.504(b)(1)(ii).

26. 17 C.F.R. § 230.504(b)(1)(iii).

27. 17 C.F.R. §§ 230.505(a), 505(b)(1). The $5 million includes (1) the securities involved in the issue and (2) all other securities sold by the joint venture during the 12 months preceding conclusion of the offering at issue. 17 C.F.R. § 230.505(b)(2)(i).

28. 17 C.F.R. § 230.505(b)(2)(iii).

29. 17 C.F.R. § 230.505(b)(2)(ii).

30. 17 C.F.R. § 230.501(e), cross-referenced in 17 C.F.R. § 230.505(b)(2)(i).

31. 17 C.F.R. § 230.501(e), cross-referenced in 17 C.F.R. § 230.505(b)(2)(i).

32. 17 C.F.R. § 230.501(e), cross-referenced in 17 C.F.R. § 230.505(b)(2)(i).

33. 17 C.F.R. § 230.502(c), cross-referenced in 17 C.F.R. § 230.505(b)(1).

34. 17 C.F.R. § 230.502(b)(1), cross-referenced in 17 C.F.R. § 230.506(b)(1).

35. 17 C.F.R. § 230.502(b)(2), cross-referenced in 17 C.F.R. § 230.506(b)(1).

36. 17 C.F.R. § 230.502(b)(2), cross-referenced in 17 C.F.R. § 230.506(b)(1).

37. 17 C.F.R. § 230.502(b)(1), cross-referenced in 17 C.F.R. § 230.505(b)(1).

38. 17 C.F.R. § 230.502(b)(1), cross-referenced in 17 C.F.R. § 230.505(b)(1).

39. 17 C.F.R. § 230.501(d), cross-referenced in 17 C.F.R. § 230.505(b)(1).

40. 17 C.F.R. § 230.502(d), cross-referenced in 17 C.F.R. § 505(b)(1). The SEC recognizes that there may be other methods by which to exercise reasonable care to ensure any transfer or resale of the securities comports with the requirements of or exception to the Securities Act. 17 C.F.R. § 230.503(d).

41. 17 C.F.R. § 230.506(b).

42. 17 C.F.R. § 230.506(b)(2)(ii).

43. 17 C.F.R. § 230.502(h), cross-referenced in 17 C.F.R. § 230.506(b)(2)(ii).

44. 17 C.F.R. § 230.506(b)(2)(ii).

45. 15 U.S.C. § 77(6). Section 4(6) creates an exemption from the registration requirements of §§ 5 and 3(a)(11) of the Securities Act but does not create an exemption to the antifraud, civil liability, or other provisions in the Act.

46. See supra note 22 in this chapter and accompanying text.

47. 15 U.S.C. § 77d(d).

48. 17 C.F.R. Part 230, Subpart 5, Preliminary Note 3.

49. The following companies are excluded from relying upon Regulation A: (1) companies required to file certain reports under the Exchange Act, (2) most foreign issuers, (3) development companies formed with no business purpose or only to merge with other entities, (4) companies issuing certain oil, gas, or mineral rights, and (5) companies subject to certain sanctions involving federal securities laws. 17 C.F.R. § 230.251(a).

50. 17 C.F.R. § 230.251(b).

51. 17 C.F.R. § 230.251(b).

52. 17 C.F.R. §§ 230.251(d)(1), 230.252-230.254.

53. 17 C.F.R. § 230.251(d)(1).

54. 17 C.F.R. § 230.251(d)(2)(i). If a preliminary (rather than a final) circular is delivered prior to the sale, a final circular must be delivered to the purchaser with the confirmation of sale. 17 C.F.R. § 230.251(d)(2)(i).

55. 17 C.F.R. § 230.251(b).

56. See 15 U.S.C. §§ 77, 781(a) (generally requiring companies issuing securities on a national exchange to register under the Exchange Act), 781(g)(1) (generally requiring companies to register under the Exchange Act if their securities are held by 500 or more people and certain other requirements are met), 78m(a) (limiting the obligation to publish periodic and other reports to those entities with securities registered under the Exchange Act), 15 U.S.C. § 78o(d) (limiting the obligation to publish similar reports to those entities which have registered securities under the Securities Act).

57. 15 U.S.C. § 78o(d) (limiting the obligation to publish similar reports to those entities that have registered securities under the Securities Act).

CHAPTER 6

Medicare Certification and Enrollment

INTRODUCTION

Joint ventures furnishing clinical services to patients might wish to participate in federal health care programs such as Medicare, Medicaid, Tricare, and the Federal Employees Health Benefits Plan ("FEHBP"). Medicaid participation requirements are codified in state law, and participation in Tricare and FEHBP is negotiated by contract. Participation in Medicare, however, requires compliance with a number of federal statutory and regulatory requirements.

GENERAL PROVISIONS

The Medicare enrollment and certification requirements vary depending upon the type of clinical joint venture. Requirements applicable to the most common types of clinical joint ventures are described below.

APPLICATION TO HOSPITAL JOINT VENTURES

Joint Venture Hospitals

The precise certification requirements associated with a hospital joint venture will vary depending upon whether the hospital is a new or existing and operational facility.

New Hospital

If the hospital is new, it must undergo full certification prior to commencing participation in the Medicare program. This involves three principal steps.

Submission of Enrollment Application The joint venture must submit a completed version of the CMS Form 855A to the Medicare fiscal intermediary of its choice and furnish informal notice of its actions to the appropriate state agency responsible for licensing the new facility ("State Survey Agency").[1] The fiscal intermediary will verify information in the enrollment form and likely ask for additional information pertinent to its review.[2] The Form 855A must be submitted under the signature and certification of a member or officer duly authorized by the joint venture to secure enrollment in the Medicare program and bind the joint venture to comply with program policies and procedures.[3] The Form will include disclosures relating to:

- Services to be provided, practice locations, tax status, and corporate form of the applicant.[4]

- Licenses and permits.[5]

- Adverse legal action and overpayments involving the applicant (under its current or a former name or business identity), those persons maintaining a 5% or greater ownership interest in the applicant, those persons with managing control in the applicant, or those persons maintaining a partnership interest in the applicant.[6]

- The billing and claims-submission service (if any) to be used by the applicant.[7]

The joint venture must also concurrently submit a CMS Form 855B (involving similar disclosures) to the local Medicare carrier in order to secure one or more Medicare Part B billing numbers.[8] CMS has recently issued a formal proposal reserving its right to conduct on-site inspection to validate disclosures made in enrollment applications.[9] Knowing and willful falsifications on a Form 855A or 855B can result in imprisonment, criminal fines, civil penalties, financial assessments, common law claims, and exclusion from the Medicare program.[10] CMS has proposed to require facilities to revalidate their Form 855 disclosures on at least a triennial basis.[11]

Survey and Certification Once the joint venture submits the Part A enrollment application to the pertinent fiscal intermediary, it will be subject to on-site inspection for compliance with conditions of participation enumerated by the Medicare program.[12] These conditions of participation include standards relating to "basic hospital functions" (e.g., quality assurance, medical staff, nursing services, medical record services, pharmaceutical services, radiologic services, laboratory services, food and dietetic services, utilization review, physical environment, infection control, discharge planning, and organ procurement) as well as certain "optional hospital services" (e.g., surgical services, anesthesia services, nuclear medicine services, outpatient services, emergency services, rehabilitation services, and respiratory care services).[13] The hospital may either submit to on-site inspection and direct certification by the Survey Agency, or, alternatively, on-site inspection by the Joint Commission on Accreditation of Healthcare Organizations ("JCAHO") or the American Osteopathic Association ("AOA"), and indirect certification through accreditation by either organization.[14] CMS has concluded that the accreditation standards promulgated by JCAHO and AOA are sufficiently rigorous that any hospital accredited by either of these organizations is thereby deemed to comply with the applicable Medicare conditions of participation.[15] Nonetheless, CMS tasks Survey Agencies to periodically conduct validation surveys of a small number of accredited institutions to ensure that institutions receiving accreditation do, in fact, comport with the Medicare conditions of participation.[16] The hospital must be licensed and operating at the time of the survey or accreditation inspection.[17]

Provider Agreement Once the State Survey Agency or accreditation organization determines that a hospital is operated in compliance with the Medicare conditions of participation, it will forward its recommendation of certification to the pertinent CMS regional office. If the regional office concurs with the recommendation, it will submit a provider agreement for execution by the facility representative designated in the Form 855A.[18] The agreement requires the provider to do all of the following:

- Observe certain civil rights requirements (including, without limitation, those promulgated under the Civil Rights Act of 1964, the Rehabilitation Act of 1973, the Age Discrimination Act of 1975).

- Satisfy certain requirements relating to advance directives.

- Abide by certain limits in charging beneficiaries for services.

- Agree to return excess cost-sharing charges to beneficiaries.

- Comply with restrictions relating to the hiring of former employees of a fiscal intermediary.

- Provide, directly or under arrangements, designated Medicare-covered services to inpatients and outpatients.

- Maintain a prescribed agreement with a Medicare Quality Improvement Organization.

- Maintain adequate admissions procedures to identify payors primary to Medicare and bill such primary payors prior to billing Medicare.

- Participate in the CHAMPUS/CHAMPVA programs.

- Admit certain veterans as directed by the Department of Veterans Affairs.

- Comply with the provisions of the Emergency Medical Treatment and Active Labor Act.

- Provide each beneficiary with a written notice at admission regarding his or her discharge rights.[19]

Once signed, the agreement is returned to CMS. If CMS concludes that the provider has disclosed all requisite information relating to provider owner- ship, none of the provider's principals have been convicted of fraud, and the provider has furnished adequate assurances that it will comply with civil rights requirements, conditions of coverage, and all other pertinent Medicare requirements, CMS will forward a signed copy of the agreement to the provider, indicating the effective date of Medicare participation.[20] The agree- ment will be deemed retroactively effective to the date when, in CMS' view, the hospital first complied with all Medicare conditions of participation (with the possible exception of certain "low-level deficiencies" for which an accept- able plan of correction has been submitted).[21] Thus, the hospital may submit claims to Medicare for services furnished to program beneficiaries as early as the effective date of the provider agreement.

Existing Hospital

If the joint venture transaction involves acquisition of an existing facility already participating in the Medicare program, the joint venture must assess (1) whether its acquisition of the hospital will constitute a change of owner- ship ("CHOW") as defined by the Medicare program, and (2) if so, whether the joint venture will accept automatic assignment of the hospital's existing Medicare provider agreement or undergo enrollment as a new Medicare provider.

In some circumstances, a joint venture member will transfer all or substan- tially all of the hospital's assets to the joint venture entity in return for its share of equity in the joint venture. In other circumstances, the joint venture will acquire substantially all of the assets of an unrelated hospital. Under either scenario, the person selling or transferring the hospital assets is oblig- ated to furnish written notice of the sale to the CMS regional office (including a copy of the purchase agreement) no later than 15 days after consummation of the transaction.[22] The regional office, with input from the Survey Agency, will, in turn, make the formal assessment as to whether a CHOW has occurred.[23] If so, the seller must file a terminating cost report for the hospital facility.[24]

Under the foregoing scenarios, the transfer will likely be deemed to constitute a CHOW for Medicare certification purposes (even when the contributing hospital maintains a substantial stake in the joint venture now deemed to own the hospital assets).[25] If a CHOW occurs, the new owners must submit a complete Form 855A, and the transferring owners must submit revised disclosures and certifications in §§ 1A-1B, 15 of a separate Form 855A formally denoting the transfer of ownership.[26] Two copies of the draft sales agreement must be included with the Form 855A submissions, followed by two copies of the final agreement once executed.[27] Additionally, the joint venture will have the choice to accept automatic assignment of the hospital's Medicare provider agreement or, alternatively, to undergo the Medicare certification process as if it were a new provider.[28]

If the joint venture accepts automatic assignment of the hospital's provider agreement, it will be subject to all terms and conditions therein, all corrective actions involving the former owner, and, with few exceptions, any penalties imposed for operation of the facility under the prior owner, as well as any claims for Medicare or Medicaid overpayments made to the prior owner.[29] If the facility is accredited, the new owner must immediately inform the accrediting organization of the CHOW, and the accrediting body will then determine whether immediate re-survey is necessary.[30]

If the new provider does not accept automatic assignment of the provider agreement, it must provide written notice to that effect to the pertinent CMS regional office.[31] Once ownership is transferred, the facility will not be eligible for Medicare reimbursement, with limited exceptions for certain emergency services.[32] The facility, however, may submit an application to be designated as a new provider in its own right in the Medicare program pursuant to the enrollment process designated for new facilities.[33] Although this strategy will result in interruption in Medicare reimbursement, it will substantially reduce the likelihood that the new ownership can be held liable for civil penalties, overpayments, corrective actions, or other liabilities of the prior owner.[34]

Joint Venture Outpatient Surgery Facilities

Joint venture outpatient surgery facilities can take either of two forms when participating in the Medicare program. If located off the hospital campus, the joint venture facility must take the form of a Medicare-certified freestanding ambulatory surgery center ("ASC"). If located on the hospital campus, the facility can take the form of an ASC or a provider-based surgery center ("PSC"). The choice of entity makes a substantial difference.

First, these two types of surgery facilities currently receive Medicare reimbursement under distinct payment systems. ASCs are reimbursed via the Medicare ASC fee schedule while PSCs are reimbursed pursuant to the hospital outpatient prospective payment system. Thus, reimbursement for a given procedure may vary between the two settings.

Second, the array of procedures covered by Medicare in the ASC context is more limited than the procedure that may be covered in a PSC.

Third, ASCs and PSCs are certified for Medicare participation through distinct processes with distinct requirements. ASCs are surveyed or accredited for compliance with distinct conditions of coverage for ASCs, subject to a distinct Medicare participation agreement from that of the hospital, utilize a distinct billing number from that of the hospital and are not carried on the hospital's cost report. PSCs are surveyed or accredited as part of the hospital for compliance with the conditions of participation applicable to hospitals, are subject to the hospital's provider agreement, are carried on the hospital's cost report, and utilize a billing number issued to the hospital.

Finally, ASCs and PSCs are treated differently under the Stark Law. As noted above, most ASC services are not designated health services implicating the Stark Law. Thus, a physician maintaining a financial relationship with an ASC is permitted to refer Medicare patients to the ASC for ASC services. By contrast, services furnished by a PSC (i.e., outpatient hospital services) are designated services that implicate the Stark Law. Thus, a physician maintaining a financial relationship with a PSC joint venture will be prohibited from referring Medicare patients there, absent an applicable Stark Law exception.

Based on the foregoing information, the joint venture will determine whether to structure its surgery facility as an ASC or PSC. Each option is presented in turn.

ASC

New ASC

Survey and Certification

Prior to submission of the enrollment application, the ASC will be subject to on-site inspection for compliance with conditions of coverage enumerated by the Medicare program.[35] These conditions of participation include standards relating to each of the following:

- Compliance with state licensure law.
- Governing body and management.
- Surgical services.

- Evaluation of quality.

- Environment.

- Medical staff.

- Nursing services.

- Medical records.

- Pharmaceutical services.

- Laboratory services.

- Radiological services.[36]

The inspection may take one of three forms. If CMS determines that the relevant state licensure requirements are at least as rigorous as the Medicare conditions of coverage, CMS will deem a facility with state licensure to be compliant with the applicable conditions of coverage. In other states, an ASC has two options. It may submit to direct inspection by the state Survey Agency for compliance with the Medicare conditions of coverage or, alternatively, to on-site inspection by an accreditation agency whose standards have been deemed by CMS to be at least as rigorous as the conditions of coverage.[37] CMS has concluded that the accreditation standards promulgated by JCAHO, AAHC, and AAAASF are sufficiently rigorous that any ASC accredited by them will be deemed to comply with the applicable Medicare conditions of coverage.[38] Nonetheless, CMS tasks Survey Agencies to conduct periodic validation surveys of a small number of accredited ASCs to ensure that they do, in fact, comport with the Medicare conditions of coverage.[39]

Enrollment

If the joint venture is opening a new ASC or converting a PSC into an ASC, it must submit a completed version of the CMS Form 855B to the local Medicare carrier and should furnish notice of its actions to the Survey Agency.[40] The carrier will verify information in the enrollment form and likely ask for additional information pertinent to its review.[41] Form 855A must be submitted under the signature and certification of a member or officer duly authorized by the joint venture to secure enrollment in the Medicare program and bind the joint venture to comply with program policies and procedures.[42] The Form will include disclosures relating to:

- Accreditation.[43]

- Services to be provided, practice locations, tax status and corporate form of the applicant.[44]

- Adverse legal action and overpayments involving the applicant (under its current or a former name or business identity), those persons maintaining a 5% or greater ownership interest in the applicant, those persons managing control of the applicant, or those persons maintaining a partnership interest in the applicant.[45]

- The billing and claims-submission service (if any) to be used by the applicant.[46]

CMS has recently issued a formal proposal reserving its right to conduct on-site inspection to validate disclosures made in enrollment applications.[47] Knowing and willful falsifications on a Form 855B can result in imprisonment, criminal fines, civil penalties, financial assessments, common law claims, and exclusion from the Medicare program.[48] CMS has proposed to require facilities to revalidate their Form 855 disclosures on at least a triennial basis.[49]

Supplier Agreement

Once the State Survey Agency or accreditation organization determines that an ASC is operated in compliance with the Medicare conditions of participation, it will forward its recommendation of certification to the pertinent CMS regional office. If the regional office concurs with the findings and has received a complete enrollment application, it will submit a provider agreement for execution by the facility representative designated in the Form 855B.[50] The agreement requires the provider to:

- Meet the Medicare conditions of coverage pertinent to ASCs (and immediately report to CMS failure to do so).

- Limit cost-sharing charges imposed upon Medicare beneficiaries.

- Promptly return cost-sharing amounts incorrectly collected from Medicare beneficiaries.

- Furnish cost information to CMS for use in calculating ASC reimbursement rates.

- Accept assignment for all ASC facility services furnished to Medicare beneficiaries.[51]

Once signed, the agreement is returned to CMS. If CMS concludes that the provider has disclosed all requisite information relating to provider ownership, none of the provider's principles have been convicted of fraud, and the applicant has furnished adequate assurances that it will comply with civil rights requirements, conditions of coverage, and all other pertinent Medicare requirements, CMS will forward a signed copy to the applicant, indicating the effective date of the agreement.[52]

Existing Provider If the joint venture transaction involves acquisition of an existing ASC already participating in the Medicare program, the person selling or transferring the facility is obligated to furnish written notice of the sale to the pertinent carrier and the CMS regional office (including a copy of the purchase agreement).[53] If the transaction results in the use of a new tax identification number by the ASC, the joint venture will be required to enroll in Medicare as the new operator of the ASC by submitting a complete Form CMS 855B.[54] The carrier will then contact state authorities to determine whether, under state law, the facility must be resurveyed or relicensed.[55] If so, the carrier will hold the enrollment application in abeyance pending completion of such action.[56] If resurvey or relicensure is not required under state law, the carrier will issue a supplier number to the new owner for use in billing services at the ASC.[57]

PSC

Regardless of whether a joint venture forms a new PSC on the campus of the hospital member of the joint venture ("Hospital Member") or acquires an interest in a PSC already operated by the Hospital Member on its campus, there are a number of regulatory requirements that must be met.

General Requirements First, the PSC must be operated on the main campus and under the license of the Hospital Member.[58] CMS will, however, disregard the common licensure requirement (though not the geographic location requirement) in jurisdictions in which state authorities prohibit the common licensure of a hospital and PSC.[59]

Second, the clinical services of the Hospital Member and PSC must be integrated in the following manner:

- Professional staff of the PSC must have clinical privileges at the Hospital Member's facility.

- The Hospital Member must maintain the same monitoring and oversight for the PSC as it does for any of its other clinical departments.

- The medical director of the PSC must maintain a reporting relationship to the chief medical officer of the Hospital Member, which is of the same frequency, intensity, and level of accountability as that between the chief medical officer and the medical director of any other hospital department.

- Medical staff committees and other professional committees at the Hospital Member must be responsible for medical activities at the PSC (including quality assurance, utilization review, and integration of services between the PSC and the Hospital Member).

- Medical records of those treated at the PSC must be integrated into the medical records retrieval system maintained by the Hospital Member.

- Patients treated at the PSC who require further care must have full access to all services at the Hospital Member's facility and be referred to the appropriate clinical unit of the Hospital Member.[60]

Third, the "financial operations" of the PSC must be "fully integrated" within the financial system of the Hospital Member "as evidenced by shared income and expenses and designation as a cost center on the Hospital Member's Medicare cost report."[61]

Fourth, the PSC must be described to the public and other payors as part of the Hospital Member.[62] For example, patients treated at the PSC must be made aware they are at a facility operated by the Hospital and are billed accordingly.[63]

Fifth, the PSC must satisfy health, safety, and nondiscrimination requirements binding upon the Hospital Member (e.g., billing for physician services using the facility site-of-service modifier, operation in compliance with the hospital's provider agreement, and compliance with all health and safety requirements applicable to the Hospital Member under the Medicare conditions of participation).[64]

Finally, not all patient services provided at the PSC may be furnished "under arrangements."[65]

Designation and Enrollment A joint venture facility meeting the foregoing requirements may simply bill for its services as hospital outpatient services.[66] Alternatively, the facility may have the Member Hospital submit an attestation to the pertinent fiscal intermediary and the CMS regional office indicating that the PSC meets the foregoing requirements, maintains adequate documentation to support the attestation, and will furnish such documentation to CMS upon request.[67] CMS will provide written acknowledgment that it has received the attestation and any necessary additional information and will thereafter issue a determination as to whether the facility is provider-based.[68] Theoretically, the principal benefit to the latter approach is that if CMS thereafter determines that the PSC does not qualify as provider-based, it would not seek to recoup all payments made during periods subject to re-opening, but would rather recover only the marginal difference between the amount of Medicare reimbursement which would have been paid if the facility were not provider-based.[69] This distinction may be irrelevant with respect to PSCs because most services furnished there would not qualify for reimbursement in any setting other than a PSC or ASC, and CMS has not indicated that it would equate PSCs violating provider-based status requirements with licensed and certified ASCs.[70]

Neither the Hospital Member nor the joint venture need file a new Form 855A when opening the PSC because the facility will be operated as part of the hospital. Nonetheless, § 4 of the existing Form 855A might need to be revised to reflect the address of the PSC on the hospital campus, as well as the ownership in the PSC.[71] Moreover, the joint venture must also concurrently submit a CMS Form 855B (involving similar disclosures) to the local Medicare carrier in order to secure any additional Medicare Part B billing numbers to be used at the PSC.[72]

Survey, Certification, and Provider Agreement The joint venture should inform the Survey Agency and any accreditation organization accrediting the hospital of the new facility, although an interim inspection or accreditation survey will not necessarily be required. The PSC will not execute a Medicare provider agreement, but will be subject to the Member Hospital's provider agreement.

Joint Venture Imaging Facilities

Hospitals can also participate in joint venture diagnostic imaging facilities.[73] Such arrangements are further facilitated by the fact that the Stark Law will not generally preclude radiologists from furnishing services to Medicare beneficiaries at the center.[74]

Enrollment

If the joint venture is opening a new independent imaging facility, it must enroll in the Medicare Part B program as an independent diagnostic testing facility ("IDTF") by submitting a completed version of the CMS Form 855B (including attachment 2) to the local Medicare carrier.[75] The carrier will verify information in the enrollment form and likely ask for additional information pertinent to its review.[76] The Form 855B must be submitted under the signature and certification of a member or officer duly authorized by the joint venture to secure enrollment in the Medicare program and bind the joint venture to comply with program policies and procedures.[77] Disclosures include those applicable to all Medicare suppliers as well as those required only from prospective IDTFs:

- Services to be provided, practice locations, tax status and corporate form of the applicant.[78]

- Adverse legal action and overpayments involving the applicant (under its current or a former name or business identity), those persons maintaining a 5% or greater ownership interest in the applicant, those persons with managing control of the applicant, or those persons maintaining a partnership interest in the applicant.[79]

- The billing and claims-submission service (if any) to be used by the applicant.[80]

- All CPT-4 and HCPCS codes to be billed by the facility.[81]

- Each type of equipment (including model number) that the facility will use in furnishing imaging services.[82]

- Information identifying the physicians whose diagnostic test interpretations will be billed by the facility.[83]

- Disclosure of the names and credentials of sufficiently numerous and qualified technicians to perform the designated diagnostic tests conducted at the facility.[84]

- Disclosure of the names and credentials of sufficiently numerous and qualified physician(s) supervising the tests furnished at the facility.[85]

- Certification from the supervising physician(s).[86]

- Certification that, as of the date on which the Form 855B is submitted, that Facility meets the Medicare requirements governing IDTFs.[87]

CMS has recently issued a formal proposal reserving its right to conduct on-site inspection to validate disclosures made in enrollment applications.[88] Knowing and willful falsifications on a Form 855B can result in imprisonment, criminal fines, civil penalties, and financial assessments, common law claims, and exclusion from the Medicare program.[89] CMS has proposed to require facilities to revalidate their Form 855 disclosures on at least a triennial basis.[90]

Certification

Within 60 days of receipt of the complete Form 855B, the pertinent Medicare carrier will conduct a site visit.[91] The site visit will typically be unannounced and is designed to determine whether the IDTF actually exists, whether the supervisory physician(s) and technicians designated in the enrollment application are properly credentialed and licensed and are performing their duties, and that equipment is properly maintained and calibrated.[92] The carrier will also ask to interview personnel and review written policies to determine how the facility ensures that the supervising physician furnishes the adequate level of supervision.[93] If, based upon the site visit and Form 855B disclosures, the carrier believes that the facility satisfies the requirements relating to IDTF designation, it will thereafter issue a Medicare supplier number to the IDTF.

Joint Venture Clinical Laboratories

Hospitals can also joint venture clinical laboratory facilities.[94] Such arrangements are further facilitated by the fact that pathologists investing in such a joint venture given that the Stark Law will not generally preclude the pathologists from furnishing services to Medicare beneficiaries at the facility.[95]

New Facility

CLIA Certification Before a clinical laboratory may receive Medicare reimbursement, it must first secure a certificate of compliance or certificate of accreditation. As a preliminary step, the joint venture must secure a "registration certificate" from the CMS regional office, permitting operation of the facility pending certification or accreditation.[96] Thereafter, the laboratory must either submit to survey by the Survey Agency or, alternatively, submit to an accreditation survey from an organization that CMS has deemed to impose accreditation standards at least as rigorous as those imposed by the Clinical Laboratory Improvement Act of 1988 ("CLIA").[97] Thereafter, a CLIA number and certificate of compliance or accreditation will be issued to the joint venture for the facility.[98]

Medicare Enrollment If the joint venture is opening a new clinical laboratory and desires to receive Medicare reimbursement, it must submit a completed version of the CMS Form 855B to the local Medicare carrier. The carrier will verify information in the enrollment form and likely ask for additional information pertinent to its review.[99] Form 855B must be submitted under the signature and certification of a member or officer duly authorized by the joint venture to secure enrollment in the Medicare program and bind the joint venture to comply with program policies and procedures.[100] Disclosures include:

- Services to be provided, practice locations, tax status and corporate form of the applicant.[101]

- Adverse legal action and overpayments involving the applicant (under its current or a former name or business identity), those persons maintaining a 5% or greater ownership interest in the applicant, those persons with managing control of the applicant, or those persons maintaining a partnership interest in the applicant.[102]

- The billing and claims-submission service (if any) to be used by the applicant.[103]

- CLIA and FDA certifications.[104]

CMS has recently issued a formal proposal reserving its right to conduct on-site inspection to validate disclosures made in enrollment applications.[105] Knowing and willful falsifications on a Form 855B can result in imprisonment, criminal fines, civil penalties, and financial assessments, common law claims, and exclusion from the Medicare program.[106] Upon receipt of a complete Form 855B and accompanying CLIA certification, the carrier will issue a Medicare Part B number to the joint venture for testing services furnished at the laboratory.[107] CMS has proposed to require facilities to revalidate their Form 855 disclosures on at least a triennial basis.[108]

Existing Facility

If the joint venture transaction involves acquisition of an existing clinical laboratory already participating in the Medicare program, the person selling or transferring the facility is obligated to furnish written notice of the sale to the pertinent carrier and the CMS regional office (including a copy of the purchase agreement).[109] The joint venture will be required to enroll in Medicare as the new operator of the laboratory by submitting a complete Form CMS 855B.[110] The carrier will then contact state authorities to determine whether, under state law, the facility must be resurveyed or relicensed.[111] If so, the carrier will hold the enrollment application in abeyance pending completion of such action.[112] If resurvey or relicensure is not required under state law, the carrier will issue a supplier number to the new owner for use in billing services at the laboratory.[113]

Joint Venture Rehabilitation Clinics

New Facility

If the joint venture will open a new clinic for the furnishing of outpatient physical therapy, it must undergo full certification prior to commencing participation in the Medicare program.[114] This involves a number of steps, the first of which is submission of an enrolled application.

Submission of Enrollment Application The joint venture must submit a completed version of the CMS Form 855A to the Medicare fiscal intermediary of its choice and informal notice of its actions to the Survey Agency.[115] The fiscal intermediary will verify information in the enrollment form and likely ask for additional information pertinent to its review.[116] The Form 855A must be submitted under the signature and certification of a member or officer duly authorized by the joint venture to secure enrollment in the Medicare program and bind the joint venture to comply with program policies and procedures.[117] The Form will include disclosures relating to:

- Services to be provided, practice locations, tax status and corporate form of the applicant.[118]

- Licenses and permits.[119]

- Adverse legal action and overpayments involving the applicant (under its current or a former name or business identity), those persons maintaining a 5% or greater ownership interest in the applicant, those persons with managing control of the applicant, or those persons maintaining a partnership interest in the applicant.[120]

- The billing and claims-submission service (if any) to be used by the applicant.[121]

CMS has recently issued a formal proposal reserving its right to conduct on-site inspection to validate disclosures made in enrollment applications.[122] Knowing and willful falsifications on a Form 855A can result in imprisonment, criminal fines, civil penalties, and financial assessments, common law claims, and exclusion from the Medicare program.[123] CMS has proposed to require facilities to revalidate their Form 855 disclosures on at least a triennial basis.[124]

Survey and Certification Once the Part A enrollment application has been submitted to the pertinent fiscal intermediary, it will be subject to on-site inspection for compliance with conditions of participation enumerated by the Medicare program.[125] These conditions of participation include standards relating to:

- Compliance with federal, state, and local law.

- Licensure and registration of staff.

- Administration and management.

- Maintenance of patient-specific plans of care.

- Physician involvement.

- Physical therapy services.

- Speech pathology services.

- Rehabilitation program.

- Use of contract personnel.

- Maintenance of clinical records.

- Physical environment.

- Infection control.

- Disaster preparedness.

- Program evaluation.[126]

The clinic may either submit to on-site inspection and direct certification by the Survey Agency, or, alternatively, on-site inspection by a CMS-designated accreditation agency, and deemed compliance as a result of such accreditation.[127] Nonetheless, CMS tasks Survey Agencies to periodically conduct validation surveys of small number of accredited institutions to ensure that institutions receiving accreditation do, in fact, comport with the Medicare conditions of participation.[128] The clinic must be licensed and operating at the time of the survey or accreditation inspection.[129]

Provider Agreement Once the State Survey Agency or accreditation organization determines that a hospital is operated in compliance with the Medicare conditions of participation, it will forward its recommendation of certification to the pertinent CMS regional office. If the regional office concurs with the findings, it will submit a provider agreement for execution by the facility representative designated in the Form 855A.[130] The agreement requires the provider to:

- Observe certain civil rights requirements (including, without limitation, those promulgated under the Civil Rights Act of 1964, the Rehabilitation Act of 1973, the Age Discrimination Act of 1975).

- Limit charges levied upon beneficiaries.

- Agree to return excess cost-sharing charges to the beneficiary.

- Comply with restrictions relating to the hiring of former employees of a fiscal intermediary.

- Maintain adequate admissions procedures to identify payors primary to Medicare and bill such primary payors prior to Medicare.

Once signed, the agreement is returned to CMS. If CMS concludes that the provider has disclosed all requisite information relating to provider ownership, none of the provider's principals have been convicted of fraud, and the provider has furnished adequate assurances that it will comply with civil rights requirements, conditions of coverage, and all other pertinent Medicare requirements, CMS will forward a signed copy to the provider, indicating the effective date of the agreement.[131] The agreement will be deemed retroactively effective to the date when, in CMS' view, the provider first complied with all Medicare conditions of participation (with the possible exception of certain "low-level deficiencies" for which an acceptable plan of correction has been submitted).[132] Thus, the clinic may submit claims to Medicare furnished as early as the effective date of the provider agreement.

Existing Clinic

If the joint venture transaction involves acquisition of an existing facility already participating in the Medicare program, the joint venture must assess (1) whether its acquisition of the entity will constitute a CHOW change of ownership as defined by the Medicare program, and (2) if so, whether the joint venture will accept automatic assignment of the facility's Medicare provider agreement or undergo enrollment as a new Medicare provider.

The new owners must submit a complete Form 855A and the transferring owners must submit revised disclosures and certifications in §§ 1A-1B, 15 of a separate Form 855A formally denoting the transfer of ownership.[133] Two copies of the draft sales agreement must be included with the Form 855A submissions, followed by two copies of the final agreement once executed.[134] Additionally, the joint venture will have the choice to accept automatic assignment of the entity's Medicare provider agreement or, alternatively, to undergo the Medicare certification process as if it were a new provider.[135]

In most circumstances, a joint venture member will transfer all or substantially all of the clinic's assets to the joint venture entity in return for its share of equity in the joint venture. The person selling or transferring the clinic assets is obligated to furnish written notice of the sale to the CMS regional office (including a copy of the purchase agreement) no later than 15 days after consummation of the transaction.[136] The regional office—with input from the Survey Agency—will, in turn, make the formal assessment as to whether a CHOW has occurred.[137] This transfer will likely be deemed to constitute a CHOW for Medicare certification purposes, even though the contributing provider retains a substantial stake in the joint venture now deemed to own the facility assets.[138] If so, the seller must file a terminating cost report for the clinic.[139] Thus, the joint venture will have the choice to accept automatic assignment of the facility's Medicare provider agreement or, alternatively, to undergo the Medicare certification process as if it were a new provider.[140]

If the joint venture accepts automatic assignment of the provider agreement, it will be subject to all terms and conditions therein, all corrective actions involving the former owner, and, with few exceptions, any penalties imposed for operation of the facility under the prior owner, and any claims for Medicare or Medicaid overpayments made to the prior owner.[141] If the facility is accredited, the new owner must immediately inform all relevant accrediting organizations of the CHOW, and the accrediting body will then determine whether immediate re-survey is necessary.[142] Information regarding the new owners must be submitted on a revised Form 855A.

If the new provider does not accept automatic assignment of the provider agreement, it must provide written notice to that effect to the pertinent CMS regional office.[143] Once ownership is transferred, the facility will not be eligible for Medicare reimbursement.[144] The facility, however, may submit an application to be designated a new provider in its own right in the Medicare program pursuant to the enrollment process designated for new facilities.[145] Although this strategy will result in interruption in Medicare reimbursement, it will substantially reduce the likelihood that the new ownership can be held liable for civil penalties, overpayments, corrective actions, or other liabilities of the prior owner.[146]

Joint Venture ESRD Facilities

New Facility

If the joint venture will open a new ESRD facility, it must undergo full certification prior to commencing participation in the Medicare program. This involves a number of steps.

Submission of Enrollment Application The joint venture must submit a completed version of the CMS Form 855A to the Medicare fiscal intermediary of its choice and informal notice of its actions to the Survey Agency.[147] The fiscal intermediary will verify information in the enrollment form and likely ask for additional information pertinent to its review.[148] The Form 855A must be submitted under the signature and certification of a member or officer duly authorized by the joint venture to secure enrollment in the Medicare program and bind the joint venture to comply with program policies and procedures.[149] The Form will include disclosures relating to:

- Services to be provided, practice locations, tax status and corporate form of the applicant.[150]

- Licenses and permits.[151]

- Adverse legal action and overpayments involving the applicant (under its current or a former name or business identity), those persons maintaining a 5% or greater ownership interest in the applicant, those persons with managing control of the applicant, or maintaining a partnership interest in the applicant.[152]

- The billing and claims-submission service (if any) to be used by the applicant.[153]

CMS has recently issued a formal proposal reserving its right to conduct on-site inspection to validate disclosures made in enrollment applications.[154] Knowing and willful falsifications on a Form 855A can result in imprisonment, criminal fines, civil penalties, financial assessments, common law claims, and exclusion from the Medicare program.[155] CMS has proposed to require facilities to revalidate their Form 855 disclosures on at least a triennial basis.[156]

Survey and Certification Once the Part A enrollment application has been submitted to the pertinent fiscal intermediary, it will be subject to on-site inspection for compliance with conditions of participation enumerated by the Medicare program.[157] These conditions of participation include standards relating to:

- Minimum utilization.
- Participation in CMS-designated ESRD networks.
- Compliance with federal, state, and local law.
- Governing body.
- Patient care plan.
- Patients rights and responsibilities.
- Medical records.
- Physical environment.
- Reuse of supplies.
- Affiliation agreements.
- Qualifications and duties of facility director.
- State qualifications and duties.
- Minimal service requirements.[158]

The clinic must submit to on-site inspection and direct certification by the Survey Agency.[159] The clinic must be licensed and operating at the time of the survey or accreditation inspection.[160] The clinic must also submit documentation to CMS as to how it will meet minimum utilization requirements and further the objectives of the pertinent CMS dialysis network.[161]

Supplier Approval Once the State Survey Agency or accreditation organization determines that a hospital is operated in compliance with the Medicare conditions of participation, it will forward its recommendation of certification to the pertinent CMS regional office. If the regional office concurs with the findings, it will issue a Medicare billing number to the facility.

Existing Facility

If the joint venture transaction involves acquisition of an ESRD facility already participating in the Medicare program, the joint venture must assess whether its acquisition of the facility will constitute a CHOW as defined by the Medicare program. In most circumstances, a joint venture member will transfer all or substantially all of the facility's assets to the joint venture entity in return for its share of equity in the joint venture. The person selling or transferring the facility is obligated to furnish written notice of the sale to the pertinent carrier and the CMS regional office (including a copy of the purchase agreement).[162] The regional office æ with input from the Survey Agency æwill, in turn, make the formal assessment as to whether a CHOW has occurred.[163] This transfer will likely be deemed to constitute a CHOW for Medicare certification purposes, even though the contributing entity contains a substantial stake in the joint venture now deemed to own the facility.

The new owners must submit a complete Form 855A and the transferring owners must submit revised disclosures and certifications in §§ 1A-1B, 15 of a separate for 855A formally denoting the transfer of ownership.[164] Two copies of the draft sales agreement must be included with the Form 855A submissions, followed by two copies of the final agreement once executed.[165]

ENDNOTES

1. Form CMS 855A (version dated Nov. 2001) ("Form 855A") at 3.

2. Form 855A at 3. Once the hospital is enrolled, material changes to disclosures made in Form 855A must be made within 90 days to the appropriate fiscal intermediary on an amended 855A. Form 855A at 5.

3. Form 855A at 49–55.

4. Form 855A at 15–17.

5. Form 855B at 14.

6. Form 855A at 18–19, 26–29, 33–35.

7. Form 855A at 38-41.

8. Form 855A at 14.

9. 68 Fed. Reg. 22065, 22082-22083 (2003) (proposing 42 C.F.R. § 424.510(a)(2)(ii)(E)(5)).

10. Form 855A at 47.

11. 68 Fed. Reg. at 22083 (proposing 42 C.F.R. § 424.515).

12. 42 C.F.R. § 488.3(a)(2).

13. See 42 C.F.R. Part 482, Subparts A–D. Additional requirements are prescribed for psychiatric hospitals and those acute care hospitals providing long-term-care swing bed services. 42 CFR Part 482, Subpart E.

14. 42 C.F.R. § 488.5(a). Should the joint venture choose to secure accreditation from JCAHO or AOA, it must authorize disclosure of the survey report to CMS. 42 C.F.R. § 488.5(c).

15. 42 C.F.R. § 488.5(a). Accreditation, however, does not establish compliance with the Medicare condition of participation relating to utilization review or Medicare requirements relating to staffing and medical records in psychiatric hospitals. 42 CFR § 488.5(a).

16. 42 C.F.R. § 488.7.

17. Medicare State Operations Manual § 2008 (A)-(B).

18. 42 C.F.R. § 489.11(a).

19. 42 C.F.R. § 489.10(b)-(c); 42 C.F.R. Part 489 Subpart B.

20. 42 C.F.R. §§ 489.11(c), 489.12.

21. 42 C.F.R. § 489.13(b)-(c). The retroactive period cannot exceed one year. 42 C.F.R. § 489.13(d)(2).

22. Medicare Intermediary Manual § 4501.2. See also 42 C.F.R. § 489.18(b).

23. Medicare Intermediary Manual § 4501.2; Medicare State Operations Manual § 3210.2. The pertinent fiscal intermediary will make a separate determination as to whether a CHOW occurred for reimbursement (as opposed to certification) purposes. Medicare Intermediary Manual § 4501.4. The two analyses are "similar but different." Medicare Intermediary Manual § 4501. Moreover, a CHOW can occur for purposes of Medicare certification even when a transaction does not necessarily constitute a change of ownership for purposes of state licensure. Medicare State Operations Manual § 3210.1(E).

24. Medicare Intermediary Manual § 4501.4.

25. Medicare Intermediary Manual §§ 4502.2, 4502.5; Medicare State Operations Manual § 3210.1.

26. Form 855A at 9–13.

27. Form 855A at 9.

28. 42 C.F.R. § 489.18(c); Medicare State Operations Manual § 3210.

29. 42 C.F.R. § 489.18(d); Medicare State Operations Manual § 3210. See also *Deerbrook Pavilion v. Shalala*, 235 F.3d 1100 (8th Cir. 2000) (holding that entity purchasing nursing home and accepting assignment of the nursing home's provider agreement was liable for civil money penalties imposed on nursing home prior to sale); *United States v. Vernon Home Health*, 21 F.3d 693 (5th Cir. 1994) (holding that entity purchasing assets but not liabilities of home health

agency was nonetheless jointly and severally liable for Medicare overpayments made to prior owner because the successor accepted automatic assignment of the provider agreement).

30. Medicare State Operations Manual § 3210.1(C).

31. Medicare State Operations Manual § 3210.5(A).

32. Medicare State Operations Manual § 3210.5(A).

33. Medicare State Operations Manual § 3210.5(A).

34. Liability may not be mitigated where there is substantial overlap in ownership between the entity selling and the entity purchasing the hospital's assets.

35. 42 C.F.R. § 416.26(a)-(b).

36. 42 C.F.R. §§ 416.40-416.49.

37. 42 C.F.R. § 416.26(a)-(b). Should an ASC choose to secure accreditation, it must authorize disclosure of the survey report to CMS. 42 C.F.R. § 416.26(a)(3).

38. 67 Fed. Reg. 70437 (2002); 67 Fed. Reg. 70439 (2002).

39. 42 C.F.R. § 416.26(b)(2).

40. Form CMS 855B (version dated Nov. 2001) ("Form 855B") at 3, 8.

41. Form 855B at 3. Material changes to disclosures made in Form 855B must be made within 90 days to the carrier on an amended 855B. Form 855B at 3.

42. Form 855B at 39–43.

43. Form 855B at 10.

44. Form 855B at 8–9.

45. Form 855B at 12–13, 20–29.

46. 855B at 30–33.

47. 68 Fed. Reg. at 22082-22083 (proposing 42 C.F.R. § 424.510(a)(2)(ii)(E)(5)).

48. 855B at 37.

49. 68 Fed. Reg. at 22083 (proposing 42 C.F.R. § 424.515).

50. 42 C.F.R. § 416.26(d).

51. 42 C.F.R. § 416.30.

52. 42 C.F.R. § 416.26(e).

53. Form 855B at 5. See also 42 C.F.R. § 489.18(b).

54. Program Integrity Manual Chapter 10, § 8.

55. Program Integrity Manual Chapter 10, § 8.

56. Program Integrity Manual Chapter 10, § 8.

57. Program Integrity Manual Chapter 10, § 8.

58. 42 C.F.R. §§ 413.65(d)(1), 413.65(f). For purposes of the location requirement, a Hospital Member's "campus" includes (1) the area "immediately adjacent to" the provider's main buildings, (2) structures located within 250 yards of the provider's main buildings, and (3) other areas designated at the hospital by the pertinent CMS regional office. 42 C.F.R. § 413.65(a)(2).

59. 42 C.F.R. § 413.65(d)(1).

60. 42 C.F.R. § 413.65(d)(2).

61. 42 C.F.R. § 413.65(d)(3).

62. 42 C.F.R. § 413.65(d)(4).

63. 42 C.F.R. § 413.65(d)(4).

64. 42 C.F.R. § 413.65(d)(g).

65. 42 C.F.R. § 413.65(i).

66. CMS Program Memorandum A-03-030 (April 18, 2003) at 7.

67. 42 C.F.R. § 413.65(b)(3)(i). For a description of the applicable attestation requirements, see CMS Program Memorandum A-03-030 (April 18, 2003) at 2–3.

68. 42 C.F.R. §§ 413.65(b)(3)(iii), 413.65(k).

69. CMS Program Memorandum A-03-030 at 2–3.

70. 42 C.F.R. § 413.65(k).

71. Form 855A at 5, 21, 26-29. The hospital may also be required to disclose to the fiscal intermediary its intent to secure a new Medicare Part B billing number for the PSC. Form 855A at 14.

72. Form 855A at 14.

73. Imaging facilities that furnish testing services reimbursed exclusively through the physician fee schedule are not eligible for designation as provider-based facilities. 42 C.F.R. § 413.65(a)(1)(ii)(G). Rather, they operate as freestanding facilities.

74. Even though such a radiologist would be deemed to have a "financial relationship" with the center for purposes of the Stark Law, the radiologist's furnishing of radiology services at the facility pursuant to a consultation ordered by another physician does not constitute a "referral" implicating the Law. 42 U.S.C. § 1395nn(h)(5)(C).

75. Form 855B at 3, 5, 8.

76. Form 855B at 3. Material changes to disclosures made in Form 855B must be made within ninety days to the carrier on an amended 855B. Form 855B at 3.

77. Form 855B at 39–43.

78. Form 855B at 8–9.

79. Form 855B at 12–13, 20–29.

80. Form 855B at 30–33.

81. Form 855B at 56–57.

82. Form 855B at 56–57.

83. Form 855B at 58–59. Each such physician must be enrolled in the Medicare program and have executed a reassignment of benefits. Form 855B at 58–59.

84. Form 855B at 59–60.

85. Form 855B at 564–65.

86. Form 855B at 64–65.

87. Form 855B at 56–57; 42 C.F.R. § 410.33.

88. 68 Fed. Reg. at 22082-22083 (proposing 42 C.F.R. § 424.510(a)(2)(ii)(E)(5)).

89. 855B at 37.

90. 68 Fed. Reg. at 22083 (proposing 42 C.F.R. § 424.515).

91. Program Integrity Manual Chapter 10, § 5.3.

92. Program Integrity Manual Chapter 10, § 5.3.

93. Program Integrity Manual Chapter 10, § 5.3.

94. Clinical laboratories that furnish testing services reimbursed exclusively through the physician fee schedule are not eligible for designation as provider-based facilities. 42 C.F.R. § 413.65(a)(1)(ii)(G). Rather, they operate as freestanding facilities.

95. Even though such a pathologist would be deemed to have a "financial relationship" with the center for purposes of the Stark Law, the pathologist's furnishing of pathology services at the facility pursuant to a consultation ordered by another physician does not constitute a "referral" implicating the Law. 42 U.S.C. § 1395nn(h)(5)(C).

96. State Operations Manual § 6006.

97. State Operations Manual § 6006.

98. State Operations Manual § 6006.

99. Form 855B at 3. Material changes to disclosures made in Form 855B must be made within 90 days to the carrier on an amended 855B. Form 855B at 3.

100. Form 855B at 39–43.

101. Form 855B at 8–9.

102. Form 855B at 12–13, 20–29.

103. Form 855B at 30–33.

104. Form 855B at 15, 17.

105. 68 Fed. Reg. at 22082–22083 (proposing 42 C.F.R. § 424.510(a)(2)(ii)(E)(5)).

106. Form 855B at 37.

107. Program Integrity Manual § 8.

108. 68 Fed. Reg. at 22083 (proposing 42 C.F.R. § 424.515).

109. Form 855B at 5. See also 42 C.F.R. § 489.18(b).

110. Program Integrity Manual Chapter 10, § 8.

111. Program Integrity Manual Chapter 10, § 8.

112. Program Integrity Manual Chapter 10, § 8.

113. Program Integrity Manual Chapter 10, § 8.

114. This section, focuses on a joint venture to establish a rehabilitation clinic. Medicare also covers a broad array of rehabilitation services furnished in comprehensive outpatient rehabilitation facilities ("CORFs"). These centers are far less common but face a similar

enrollment process with somewhat distinct conditions of participation. See 42 C.F.R. Part 486, Subpart B.

115. Form 855A at 3. Outpatient rehabilitation clinics are not eligible for provider-based status under the hospital outpatient prospective payment system unless/until the moratorium is lifted on the $1,500 annual cap on physical, occupational, or speech therapy. 42 C.F.R. § 413.65(a)(1)(ii)(H).

116. Form 855A at 3. Material changes to disclosures made in Form 855A must be made within 90 days to the appropriate fiscal intermediary on an amended 855A. Form 855A at 5.

117. Form 855A at 49–55.

118. Form 855A at 15–17.

119. Form 855B at 14.

120. Form 855A at 18–19, 26–29, 33–35.

121. Form 855A at 38–41.

122. 68 Fed. Reg. at 22082-22083 (proposing 42 C.F.R. § 424.510(a)(2)(ii)(E)(5).

123. Form 855A at 47.

124. 68 Fed. Reg. at 22083 (proposing 42 C.F.R. § 424.515).

125. 42 C.F.R. § 488.3(a)(2).

126. See 42 C.F.R. Part 485, subpart H.

127. 42 C.F.R. § 488.5(a).

128. 42 C.F.R. § 488.7.

129. Medicare State Operations Manual § 2008 (A)-(B).

130. 42 C.F.R. § 489.11(a).

131. 42 C.F.R. §§ 489.11(c), 489.12.

132. 42 C.F.R. § 489.13(b)-(c). The retroactivity period cannot exceed one year. 42 C.F.R. § 489.13(d)(2).

133. Form 855A at 9–13.

134. Form 855A at 9.

135. 42 C.F.R. § 489.18(c); Medicare State Operations Manual § 3210.

136. Medicare Intermediary Manual § 4501.2. See also 42 C.F.R. § 489.18(b).

137. Medicare Intermediary Manual § 4501.2; Medicare State Operations Manual § 3210.2. A CHOW can occur for purposes of Medicare certification even when a transaction does not necessarily constitute a change of ownership for purposes of state licensure. Medicare State Operations Manual § 3210.1(E).

138. Medicare Intermediary Manual §§ 4502.2, 4502.5; Medicare State Operations Manual § 3210.1.

139. Medicare Intermediary Manual § 4501.4.

140. 42 C.F.R. § 489.18(c); Medicare State Operations Manual § 3210.

141. 42 C.F.R. § 489.18(d); Medicare State Operations Manual § 3210. See also *Deerbrook Pavilion v. Shalala*, 235 F.3d 1100 (8th Cir. 2000) (holding that entity purchasing nursing home

and accepting assignment of the nursing home's provider agreement was liable for civil money penalties imposed on nursing home prior to sale); *United States v. Vernon Home Health*, 21 F.3d 693 (5th Cir. 1994) (holding that entity purchasing assets but not liabilities of home health agency was nonetheless jointly and severally liable for Medicare overpayments made to prior owner because the successor accepted automatic assignment of the provider agreement).

142. Medicare State Operations Manual § 3210.1(C).

143. Medicare State Operations Manual § 3210.5(A).

144. Medicare State Operations Manual § 3210.5(A).

145. Medicare State Operations Manual § 3210.5(A).

146. Liability may not be mitigated where there is substantial overlap in ownership between the entity selling and the entity purchasing the facility's assets.

147. Form 855A at 3. ESRD facilities cannot qualify for provider-based status for payment pursuant to the hospital outpatient prospective payment system. 42 C.F.R. § 413.65(a)(1)(ii)(I). Fiscal intermediaries do, however, certify ESRD facilities as hospital-based or freestanding under distinct (but similar) criteria for purposes of calculating the applicable reimbursement rate for the facility. 42 C.F.R. § 413.174. Unlike with the general provider-based standards for outpatient facilities, however, it is unclear whether a joint venture facility could ever qualify for provider-based status under the distinct criteria applicable to ESRD facilities.

148. Form 855A at 3. Material changes to disclosures made in Form 855A must be made within 90 days to the appropriate fiscal intermediary on an amended 855A. Form 855A at 5.

149. Form 855A at 49–55.

150. Form 855A at 15–17.

151. Form 855B at 14.

152. Form 855A at 18–19, 26–29, 33–35.

153. Form 855A at 38–41.

154. 68 Fed. Reg. at 22082–22083 (proposing 42 C.F.R. § 424.510(a)(2)(ii)(E)(5)).

155. Form 855A at 47.

156. 68 Fed. Reg. at 22083 (proposing 42 C.F.R. § 424.515).

157. 42 C.F.R. § 488.3(a)(2).

158. See 42 C.F.R. Part 405, subpart U.

159. 42 C.F.R. § 488.5(a); State Operations Manual § 2278. No accreditation agency has been granted deemed status by CMS to presumptively determine whether a facility complies with the requisite Medicare conditions of participation.

160. Medicare State Operations Manual § 2008 (A)-(B).

161. 42 C.F.R. § 488.60.

162. Form 855B at 5. See also 42 C.F.R. § 489.18(b).

163. Medicare State Operations Manual § 3210.2. A CHOW can occur for purposes of Medicare certification even when a transaction does not necessarily constitute a change of ownership for purposes of state licensure. Medicare State Operations Manual § 3210.1(E).

164. Form 855A at 9–13.

165. Form 855A at 9.

CHAPTER 7

Selecting Investors

INTRODUCTION

The manner in which investors are selected for the joint venture and the relationship of these investors to the investing hospital can raise significant compliance concerns under federal fraud and abuse law, tax law, antitrust law, and securities law. This chapter addresses the pertinent compliance concerns in each of the foregoing areas and suggests possible safeguards in the investor-selection process so as to promote compliance with federal law.

FRAUD AND ABUSE COMPLIANCE

Anti-Kickback Law

The Government's Concern

One of the OIG's "major concerns" in evaluating joint venture arrangements is that "distributions from the joint venture may, in fact, be disguised remuneration" paid to induce the generation of Federal Program business for the joint venture or joint venture investors, rather than a return-on-investment capital placed at risk to finance a legitimate business venture.[1] Under such circumstances, the OIG is concerned that joint venture distributions could lead to "overutilization" of items reimbursed by Federal Programs, "increased costs" for Federal Programs, "corruption of professional judgement" and "unfair competition" among healthcare providers.[2] Thus, the OIG's concern with "the manner in which investors are selected and retained"[3] will be limited to joint ventures in which some or all debt or equity investors are in a position to:

- Make or influence patient referrals to the joint venture or other investors for items or services which may be reimbursable by a Federal Program.[4]

141

- Generate business for the joint venture or other investors, which is reimbursable by a Federal Program.[5]

- Furnish items or services to the joint venture or other investors, which are reimbursable by a Federal Program.[6]

If those solicited for joint venture participation (either as equity or debt holders) fall into one or more of the foregoing categories, safeguards can be adopted to (1) protect the joint venture arrangement under an Anti-Kickback Law safe harbor or (2) otherwise minimize the risk that the OIG would perceive joint venture returns as a pretext for impermissible remuneration (rather than a legitimate return on capital placed at genuine risk to finance the venture).

Safe Harbor Protection

Investment Interests Generally As noted in Chapter 2, distributions from a joint venture to investors (whether equity or debt holders) can be protected under the Anti-Kickback Law so long as the joint venture maintains "strict compliance" with all requirements of the Investment Interests Safe Harbor.[7] Six of the eight Safe Harbor requirements are specifically intended to ensure safe harbor protection is afforded only when investment opportunity is broadly diffused beyond potential sources of Federal Program business for the joint venture or fellow investors and that investment returns constitute a payment for capital that the investor places at genuine risk to finance the joint venture.

First, safe harbor protection is afforded only if no more than 40% of the value of each class of investment interests in the joint venture was held in the previous fiscal year or previous 12-month period by investors who were in a position to make or influence referrals to, furnish items or services to, or otherwise generate business for the joint venture ("Business Source Investors").[8] This requirement is designed to ensure that Business Source Investors "are not in a position to dominate the joint venture's business."[9] The provision also ensures that profit distributions will be diffused to a wider group than the Business Source Investors, thereby reducing the financial incentive they might otherwise have to overutilize joint venture services or indiscriminately steer patients to the joint venture.[10]

A hospital will presumptively be deemed to be a Business Source Investor, and therefore count against the 40% limitation.[11] There is contradictory guidance as to whether a hospital can exempt itself from counting against the 40% limitation by executing (and abiding by) a written stipulation adopting operational restrictions that preclude it from generating business (including the furnishing of items or services) for the joint venture during the life of the investment.[12] As noted below, however, even if such a stipulation will not permit complete safe harbor protection, if combined with compliance with all other safe harbor requirements, it will greatly minimize the risk of an enforcement action and can lead to full protection through a favorable advisory opinion.

At their option, joint venture representatives may combine distinct but "equivalent classes" of investment interests in calculating compliance with the 40% limitation.[13] Classes of investments will be deemed to be "equivalent" so as to permit aggregation only if (1) they "have similar rights with respect to the entity's income and assets," (2) investors receive equivalent returns in proportion to the amounts invested, and (3) there is no preferential treatment of referral source investors (including, but not limited to, preferences that take effect in the event of a disposition of the entity's assets.).[14] The fact that one class of securities is held by passive investors (e.g., limited partners and limited liability company members who have not contractually agreed to assume liability for joint venture debts) and another class of securities is held by active investors (e.g., general partners or limited partners and LLC members who contractually assume liability for the joint venture's debts) does not preclude qualification as "equivalent" classes so long as the foregoing requirements are met.[15] A class of equity investments, however, can never be deemed equivalent to a class of debt investments.[16]

Second, the terms on which a joint venture investment interest is offered to a passive investor who would qualify as a Business Source Investor must be no different from the terms offered to other passive investors.[17] This provision is designed to preclude protection for joint venture arrangements involving "discriminatory marketing strategies that result in the offer of better deals" to those passive investors who qualify as Business Source Investors.[18] As noted above, a "passive investor" is (1) one who owns a debt interest, limited partnership interest, limited liability company membership interest, or a shareholder interest in an entity and (2) has not, by operation of law or written agreement, assumed liability for joint venture liabilities beyond his or her investment interest.[19] One can also be a passive investor through ownership of a passive interest in an entity that serves as an active investor in a joint venture.[20]

Third, the terms on which an investment interest is offered to a Business Source Investor must not be related to the previous or expected volume of referrals from, items or services furnished by, or business otherwise generated by that investor for the joint venture.[21] This provision is designed to preclude safe harbor protection where Business Source Investors receive investment terms that vary depending upon the volume or value of the business they can or do generate.[22]

Fourth, neither the joint venture nor joint venture investors may require that any passive investors generate business or be in a position to generate business for the joint venture as a condition for retaining an investment interest in the venture.[23] This provision will preclude safe harbor protection for arrangements in which an investor is divested of his or her investment interest if he or she fails to generate sufficient business for the joint venture, leaves the state, loses clinical privileges, and so forth.[24]

Fifth, neither the joint venture nor any investor (or person acting on behalf of the joint venture or investor) may loan funds to or guarantee a loan for a Business Source Investor if the proceeds are used in whole or part to obtain the investment interest in the joint venture.[25] This provision is designed to ensure that the investor's funds are "genuinely at risk" in the joint venture.[26] The provision does not, however, preclude the joint venture from borrowing funds from one or more investors to cover capital or operating expenses.[27]

Finally, distributions must be paid out to each investor and made in direct proportion to the amount of the investor's capital contribution (including the fair market value of pre-operational services may constitute a capital contribution).[28]

Joint ventures meeting the foregoing requirements are eligible for protection under the Investment Interests Safe Harbor so long as the remaining safe harbor requirements relating to joint venture operations are satisfied.[29]

Investment Interests in an ASC The OIG's "chief concern" regarding ASC joint ventures is similar to its concern with other types of joint venture arrangements: "a return on an investment in an ASC might be disguised as a payment for referrals" or other Federal Program business.[30] For example, a primary care physician might be offered an investment interest in an ASC "as an incentive to refer patients to the surgeon owners of the ASC."[31] The OIG has concluded that the risk of such abuse is negligible if the ASC joint venture is structured in accord with the Investment Interest Safe Harbor.[32] Under such circumstances, the risk of abuse is minimized in substantial part because the majority of the joint venture equity is held by non-Business Source investors and the majority of joint venture revenues come from noninvestors.[33]

The OIG, however, has also concluded that the risk of fraud and abuse is sufficiently low that safe harbor protection is warranted for distributions from an ASC joint venture in the alternative circumstance that the facility is so thoroughly integrated with the medical practice of its physician investors that the ASC effectively serves as an "extension of" each physician investor's office practice."[34]

Five of the nine ASC Safe Harbor requirements are specifically designed to ensure that investors (1) are either not Business Source Investors or are physicians for whom the ASC serves as an extension of their office practice and (2) receive distributions proportionate to the amount of capital that they place at legitimate risk to finance the joint venture.

First, any hospital investing in the ASC must not be in a position to make or influence referrals directly or indirectly to any investor or the ASC joint venture itself.[35] For purposes of this requirement, hospitals holding investment interests will presumptively be deemed to be in a position to generate Federal Program business to the ASC (i.e., qualify as Business Source Investors), thereby precluding safe harbor protection.[36] The OIG has suggested that a hospital can remain in compliance with the Safe Harbor provisions by executing (and abiding by) a written stipulation adopting operational restrictions that preclude it from generating business (including the furnishing of items or services) for the joint venture or fellow investors during the life of the investment.[37] In practice, the OIG has failed to accept even the most stringent restrictions on hospital interaction with the ASC or its investors as sufficient to warrant Safe Harbor protection.[38] As noted below, however, even if such a stipulation will not trigger complete safe harbor protection, if combined with compliance with all other Safe Harbor requirements, it will greatly minimize the risk of an enforcement action and can lead to full protection through a favorable advisory opinion.[39]

Second, the nonhospital ASC joint venture investors who are employed by the joint venture or any joint venture investor or otherwise qualify as Business Source Investors must collectively fall into one of the following categories:[40]

- They are all general surgeons, group practices of general surgeons, surgeons of the same specialty, or group practices of the same specialty and one-third of each surgeon investor's "medical practice income" from all sources in the prior fiscal year or 12 months was derived from ASC-Approved Procedures.[41]

- They are all physicians in the same "medical practice specialty" or groups of physicians in the same medical practice specialty, and one-third of each physician investor's "medical practice income" from all sources in the prior fiscal year or 12 months was derived from ASC-Approved Procedures.[42]

- They are all physicians in a position to refer patients to the ASC joint venture and perform procedures on such referred patients or group practices composed of such physicians and both of the following conditions are met: (1) one-third of each physician investor's "medical practice income" from all sources in the prior fiscal year or 12 calendar months was derived from ASC-Approved Procedures and (2) one-third of the ASC-Approved Procedures performed by each physician investor in the previous fiscal year or previous 12 months was performed at the ASC joint venture.[43]

Third, the terms on which an investment interest in the ASC joint venture is offered to an investor is not related to the previous or expected volume of referrals, services furnished, or the amount of business otherwise generated from the investor to the ASC.[44]

Fourth, neither the joint venture nor any investor (or person acting on behalf of the joint venture or investor) loans funds to or guarantees a loan for a Business Source Investor if the proceeds are used in whole or part to obtain the investment interest.[45] So long as this requirement is observed, the OIG believes that it is more likely that (1) joint venture investors have truly made a "substantial financial investment" and (2) distributions made to them are, in fact, a legitimate investment return for capital placed at risk.[46]

Finally, distributions must be paid out to each investor in direct proportion to the amount of capital he or she has contributed to the joint venture. For purposes of this requirement, the fair market value of pre-operational services may constitute a capital contribution.[47]

Joint ventures meeting the foregoing requirements are eligible for protection under the ASC Safe Harbor so long as the remaining safe harbor requirements relating to joint venture operations are met.[48]

Ways To Lower Risk

Investment Interests Generally There are numerous safeguards that an entity can apply when selecting potential investors and securing financing which, while not affording safe harbor protection to the investment arrangement, will nonetheless reduce the risk of fraud and abuse in the eyes of the OIG. In general, such safeguards should be designed to achieve four objectives.

First, safeguards should be adopted to ensure that a substantial portion of joint venture investors are "Independent Investors" (i.e., not Business Source Investors in a position to generate business for, furnish items or services to, or refer patients to the joint venture or fellow joint venture investors). Such a limitation will help establish that the joint venture is not controlled or dominated by Business Source Investors. Moreover, the presence of a substantial number of Independent Investors with a claim on joint venture distributions will dilute the return that each Business Source Investor would receive on referrals or other Federal Program business he or she generates for the joint venture.[49] This, in turn, should minimize the incentive to overutilize joint venture services or steer patients to the joint venture rather than more cost-effective providers.

As noted above, the mere fact that an investor is a juridical entity does not grant it status as an Independent Investor. Rather, such an investor will be deemed to be a Business Source Investor if it (1) furnishes items or services or generates patient referrals for the joint venture or fellow investors or (2) encourages its employees, contractors, or other affiliated persons to do so.

The OIG has shown a predisposition to deem an investor to be an Independent Investor even though he or she is in a position to refer patients, furnish items services, or generate business for the joint venture or fellow investors if such investor signs (and abides by) a written stipulation that he or she will refrain from doing so for the life of his or her investment interest. Additionally, the OIG has acknowledged that certain types of practitioners (e.g., radiologists and pathologists) are less likely to be in a position to generate business for, furnish items or services to, or make patient referrals to the joint venture or fellow investors (although they still likely count as Business Source Investors if they furnish items or services to the joint venture or fellow investors).[50]

Second, safeguards should be adopted to ensure that the terms on which joint venture interests are offered to (or may be retained by) investors do not vary based upon their ability to make patient referrals to, furnish items or services to, or generate business for the joint venture or joint venture investors.[51]

Third, safeguards should be adopted to ensure that each Business Source Investor directly makes a substantial capital investment in the joint venture, placing his or her capital at legitimate risk.[52] For example, neither the joint venture nor any investor (or person acting on behalf of the joint venture or investor) should loan funds to or guarantee a loan for a Business Source Investor if the proceeds are to be used in whole or part to obtain the investment interest.[53]

Finally, investment distributions paid to a given investor should be directly proportionate to the amount of capital the investor has placed at risk in the joint venture. The OIG will likely look with great suspicion upon any joint venture arrangement in which distributions are not tied directly to the amount of one's contributed capital. When pre-operational services are deemed to constitute a portion of an investor's capital contributions, affirmative steps should be taken to document the fair market value of such services and ensure it is equivalent to the equity stake provided in return. The OIG has shown some willingness to permit distributions to vary among investors based upon their respective equity holdings (as opposed to capital actually invested) so long as any variance in the amount of equity provided in return for a given capital contribution is documented to reflect a change in valuation of the joint venture at the time the capital contribution is made.[54]

Investment Interests in an ASC A joint venture to own and operate an ASC can be structured in accord with the foregoing safeguards so as to reduce the associated regulatory risk. If, however, the joint venture must include substantial ownership from Business Source Investors, an alternative approach can be taken. Specifically, safeguards can be adopted to ensure that Business Source Investors are limited to physicians who will utilize the ASC as an "extension of their office."

First, investment interests held by Business Source Investors should be limited to those who (1) are physicians and (2) derive a substantial part of their income from ASC-Approved Procedures. As noted above, the OIG believes that investment by such physicians poses less risk of fraud and abuse and is more likely driven by a desire to control their working environment, obtain accountability from staff, and so forth.[55] If the joint venture investment interest is held by a partnership, limited liability company, or other juridical entity, the OIG will assess whether each investor in that entity meets the foregoing requirements.[56]

Second, if the center will be a multispecialty ASC, further safeguards should be adopted to minimize the risk of investors engaging in cross-referrals between medical specialties. This can be accomplished by having physician investors execute and abide by a written stipulation preventing such referrals or by ensuring that each physician investor performs a substantial percentage of his or her ASC-Approved Procedures at the joint venture ASC. Again, if the joint venture investment interest is held by a partnership, limited liability company, or other juridical entity, the OIG will assess whether each investor in that entity meets the foregoing requirements.[57]

Third, precautions should be taken to address the OIG's concern that the investing hospital will leverage its relationship with employee, contract, and staff physicians to generate business for the ASC. The OIG has indicated that its concern in this regard will be minimized where the investing hospital agrees in writing that it will (1) not track referrals to the joint venture or joint venture investors, (2) neither compensate nor encourage staff or employed physicians to refer patients to the joint venture or joint venture investors, and (3) inform staff and employed physicians of these policies in writing no less than annually.[58]

Fourth, neither the joint venture nor any investor (or person acting on behalf of the joint venture or investor) should loan funds to or guarantee a loan for a Business Source Investor, if the proceeds are to be used in whole or part to obtain the investment interest.[59] As noted above, such a safeguard is particularly important to ensure the OIG that (1) joint venture investors have truly made a "substantial financial investment" and (2) distributions made to them are, in fact, a legitimate investment return for capital placed at risk.[60]

Finally, investment distributions paid to a given investor should be directly proportionate to the amount of capital the investor has placed at risk in the joint venture. The OIG will likely look with great suspicion upon any joint venture arrangement in which distributions are not tied directly to the amount of one's contributed capital. When pre-operational services are deemed to constitute a portion of an investor's capital contributions, affirmative steps should be taken to document the fair market value of such services and ensure they are equivalent to the equity stake provided in return. The OIG has shown some willingness to permit distributions to vary among investors based upon their respective equity holdings (as opposed to capital actually invested) so long as any variance in the amount of equity provided in return for a given capital contribution is documented to reflect a change in valuation of the joint venture at the time the capital contribution is made.[61]

Stark Law

Many joint ventures are conceived with the intention that physicians or other health care providers who employ, contract, or otherwise compensate physicians will take equity in or secured debt from the venture. Prior to determining whether to solicit investment from these sources or identifying which physicians or providers to solicit for participation, joint venture representatives must be cognizant of the effect that such participation would have upon the ability of the investing physician to refer Medicare patients requiring DHS to (1) the joint venture itself, (2) fellow investors (including an investing hospital, physician, or other health care provider), (3) health care providers compensating the joint venture. The effect of the Stark Law in limiting such referrals is discussed in Chapter 8.

Exclusion

HHS has discretion to exclude any entity from participation in a Federal Program if a person owning 5% or greater ownership or control interest has been (1) convicted of certain enumerated crimes relating to health care billing, patient abuse, substance abuse, or obstruction of a state or federal investigation, (2) held liable for civil monetary penalties under the Social Security Act, or (3) excluded from participation in a Federal Program.[62] Thus, joint ventures directly or indirectly involved in the furnishing of health care services must screen potential investors and periodically screen current investors for Federal Program exclusion. Moreover, the terms of any investment interest should be structured so as to (1) require the investor to immediately inform the joint venture if he/she/it is excluded from a Federal

Program and (2) permit the joint venture to immediately buy back the investment interest held by the excluded person.

TAX COMPLIANCE

To the extent that the hospital participating in a joint venture is tax-exempt under § 501(c)(3) of the Internal Revenue Code, selection of additional investors who are insiders or Disqualified Persons vis-à-vis the hospital raises the possibility that the joint venture may give rise to private inurement or Intermediate Sanctions if proper safeguards are not followed. These safeguards are discussed in Chapters 8 and 9.

ANTITRUST COMPLIANCE

Clinical Joint Ventures

If the joint venture will compete in a highly concentrated market with substantial barriers to timely market entry, joint venture equity interests should not be allotted to those competing in the same market absent an overriding business reason. If business considerations compel the distribution of joint venture equity to such competitors, the extent of their ownership in the joint venture should be kept as small as possible in order to ensure a continued incentive on the part of the investor to compete with the joint venture. Observance of such a limitation will minimize the government's antitrust concerns with the joint venture notwithstanding the fact that it operates in a market with a substantial potential for anticompetitive collusion. If joint venture representatives are aware that two or more potential investors are competitors in a highly concentrated market distinct from that in which the joint venture competes, joint venture representatives should be aware that selection of such investors might invite scrutiny from DOJ/FTC as to whether the joint venture serves as a conduit for these competitors to collude in their ongoing business operations outside the joint venture framework. Thus, joint venture equity should be distributed to such parties only for a compelling business reason.

Contract Joint Ventures

Concerns relating to selection of investor participants in a Contract Joint Venture are most salient when the joint venture will operate in one or more concentrated markets, and require that investor-members furnish their services exclusively through the Contract Joint Venture. Under such circumstances, the Joint Venture representatives should ensure that they do not maintain exclusive arrangements with such a substantial portion of the competitors in a given field as to preclude the efficient formation of a competing joint venture.[63]

SECURITIES COMPLIANCE

General

Although the Securities Act is only implicated if a joint venture offers or sells an instrument which qualifies as a "security," the term is applied with sufficient breadth by the SEC and federal courts that the venture should assume that any corporate stock, limited partnership interest, or limited liability company membership interest would be considered a security under the Act.[64] Promissory notes issued by a joint venture will also presumptively be deemed securities for purposes of the Securities Act.[65] Exceptions may apply for (1) notes executed in connection with a traditional commercial loan, (2) notes executed as part of an "open-account relationship" with a lending institution, and (3) short-term commercial paper.[66]

The Securities Act generally requires that an entity planning to offer or sell securities register them in advance with the SEC. Violation of the registration requirements of the Securities Act may subject an issuer and any individuals deemed to be promoters, to civil and criminal penalties from the SEC and to liability for rescission of the purchase price to any individual purchasing the unregistered security.[67] The registration process, however, is both expensive and time consuming. Additionally, registration may subject the joint venture to ongoing reporting and other requirements under the Securities Act and Exchange Act. Thus, joint venture representatives will most often structure their securities offerings so as to qualify for an exemption from the Securities Act registration requirements.[68]

Exemption from Registration Requirements of the Securities Act

There are a variety of bases upon which to exempt joint venture securities from the registration requirement of the Securities Act, and each focuses principally on the manner in which investors are selected.

Intrastate Offerings

When a joint venture will furnish services exclusively in the state in which it is organized and where all investors reside, the joint venture may wish to rely on the nonexclusive exemption for intrastate offerings as the principal basis for exemption from the registration requirements of the Securities Act.

Section 3(a)(11) of the Securities Act provides that the registration provisions of the Securities Act do not apply to securities that are sold by the issuer only in a single state in which it is doing business (and, if a corporation, the state in which it is incorporated and doing business) and sold only to those residing in that state.[69]

The SEC has promulgated Rule 147 as an exemption to assist issuers relying on the § 3(a)(11). Transactions complying with the exemption are assured of protection under § 3(a)(11) while transactions outside the exemption may or may not enjoy such protection.[70] In order to secure exemption status, all offers and sales made in connection with an issue of securities must comport with the exemption.[71] In order to qualify, the issuer must make all offers and sales to residents of the state in which the issuer is "resident and doing business."[72] An issuer is deemed to "reside" in the jurisdiction in which it is organized or incorporated. An issuer is deemed to be "doing business" within the state if each of the following holds true:

- 80% of its gross revenues came from rendering services in the state or the operation of a business or ownership of realty in the state.

- In the most recent semiannual fiscal period prior to the first offer in the issue, 80% of the issuer's assets were located in the jurisdiction.

- The issuer uses 80% of the net proceeds it receives from the issue in connection with the operation of a business, purchase of realty, or furnishing of services within such state or territory.

- The state is the issuer's principal place of business.[73]

For nine months after the last sale in the given issue, all resales must be made only to persons resident in the state in which the offering occurred.[74] The issuer must take a number of steps to prevent interstate resales. First, the issuer must place a legend on the securities indicating that they have not been registered under the Securities Act and cannot be sold outside the state for nine months after the last sale involving the issue.[75] Second, the issuer must issue stop transfer instructions during the nine-month period.[76] Third, the issuer must obtain a written representation from each purchaser as to its residence.[77] The issuer must provide written disclosure of the restrictions on, and the foregoing safeguards against, resale.[78]

Regulation D

If a joint venture cannot be certain that it will furnish services exclusively in the jurisdiction in which it is organized, or if it cannot raise sufficient capital from residents of that jurisdiction, it might choose to rely on one of the exemptions codified in Regulation D. Regulation D comprises three distinct exemptions from the registration requirements of the Securities Act.[79]

Offering Not Exceeding $1 Million   Nonpublicly traded entities conducting an offering that will not exceed $1 million are exempted from the registration requirements associated with the Securities Act.[80] There is no ceiling on the number of purchasers who may participate in the issue. Unlike the other Regulation D exemptions, there are neither mandated disclosures to investors prior to sale nor limits on the number of offerees.

An issuer relying on Rule 504 may not offer the securities through a "general solicitation" or "general advertising" (which includes solicitations or advertisements through periodicals, through the broadcast media, or at seminars or meetings advertised through periodicals or the broadcast media).[81] Generally, compliance with the general solicitation requirement permits offers only to persons previously known to the solicitor. Exception is made, however, in two circumstances. First, the restriction on general solicitation will not apply with respect to an issuer that offers and sells securities exclusively in a state in which the issuer (1) is required by state law to file a written disclosure statement with the state regarding the issue, (2) is required by state law to furnish such disclosure statement to investors prior to the sale of any securities from the issue, and (3) complies with these requirements.[82]

Second, the restriction will not apply with respect to an issue made in accordance with state law disclosure exemptions, which permit general solicitation and advertising regarding the issue so long as sales are made only to Accredited Investors.[83] Accredited Investors include, under certain circumstances, the following:

- Banks.

- Securities brokers and dealers registered with the SEC.

- Insurance companies.

- Investment companies registered with the SEC,

- Employee benefit plans.

- State benefit plans.

- Exempt organizations, partnerships, corporations, and business trusts maintaining over $5,000,000 in assets and not formed for purposes of acquiring the securities at issue.

- Directors, executive officers, or general partners of the issuer.

- Directors, executive officers, or general partners of a general partner of the issuer.

- Natural persons whose household net worth exceeds $1,000,000.

- Natural persons whose individual income exceeds $200,000 in each of the two most recent years and is reasonably expected to reach the same income level in the current year.

- Natural persons whose joint household income exceeds $300,000 in each of the two most recent years and is reasonably expected to reach the same income level in the current year.

- A trust with assets in excess of $5 million that was not formed for the specific purpose of acquiring the securities offered and that is directed by a "sophisticated person."

- An entity in which all equity owners are accredited investors.[84]

An issuer relying on this exemption must also take reasonable care to ensure that those purchasing securities are doing so for investment purposes and not with the intent to resell them.[85] The SEC has recognized that one method of exercising reasonable care is to (1) "make reasonable inquiry to determine the purchaser is acquiring the securities for himself or other persons," (2) make written disclosure to each purchaser prior to sale that the securities have not been registered under the Securities Act and cannot be resold absent registration or an applicable exemption from the registration requirement, and (3) placement of a legend on the document constituting the security that references restrictions on the transferability and sale of the securities.[86]

As with the requirements relating to the manner of investor solicitation, the requirements relating to resale are inapplicable under either of two circumstances. First, the restriction will not apply with respect to an issuer that (1) is required by state law to file a written disclosure statement with the state regarding the issue, (2) is required by state law to furnish such disclosure statement to investors prior to the sale of any securities from the issue, and (3) complies with these requirements.[87] Second, the restriction will not apply with respect to an issue made in accordance with state law disclosure exemptions that permit general solicitation and advertising regarding the issue so long as sales are made only to "accredited investors."[88]

Offering Not Exceeding $5 Million An entity contemplating an offering that will not exceed $5 million may qualify under Rule 505 for exemption from the registration requirements associated with the Securities Act.[89] Entities that directly or through their predecessors or affiliates, are party to (or have been sanctioned in) certain administrative or judicial proceedings relating to federal securities laws are precluded from relying upon this exception.[90]

The issuer must reasonably believe that there are no more than 35 purchasers in the offering.[91] The following purchasers, however, will not count against this limit:

- Accredited Investors.[92]

- Any Qualified Relative.[93]

- Any trust or estate in which a purchaser or any of his or her Qualified Relatives collectively own more than 50% beneficial interest.[94]

- Any organization of which a purchaser and any of his or her Qualified Relatives are beneficial owners of more than 50% of the equity securities.

An issuer relying on this exception may not offer the securities through a "general solicitation" or "general advertising" (e.g., solicitations or advertisements through periodicals, through the broadcast media, or at seminars or meetings advertised through periodicals or the broadcast media).[95] As with Rule 504 offerings, offerees must generally be known to the solicitors.

Prior to selling a security to an investor, other than an Accredited Investor, the issuer must furnish certain written materials.[96] The requisite type and scope of disclosures vary depending upon the size of the issue and type of entity issuing securities and may include audited or unaudited financial statements as well as other information.[97] Material information provided to Accredited Investors in connection with the issue must be briefly described to nonaccredited investors and made available to them upon request prior to the sale.[98] Prior to the sale, the issuer must also make available to each Nonaccredited Investor the "opportunity to ask question and receive answers concerning the terms and conditions of the offering and obtain any additional information that the issuer possesses or can acquire without unreasonable effort or expense that is necessary to verify the accuracy of the information" included in the mandatory written disclosures.[99] Written disclosure must also be provided to Nonaccredited Investors regarding the restriction on resale of the securities.[100]

An issuer relying on Rule 505 must take reasonable care to ensure that those purchasing securities are doing so for investment purposes and not with the intent to resell them.[101] The SEC has recognized that one method of exercising reasonable care is to (1) "make reasonable inquiry to determine the purchaser is acquiring the securities for himself or other persons," (2) make written disclosure to each purchaser prior to sale that the securities have not been registered under the Securities Act and cannot be resold absent registration or an applicable exemption from the registration requirement, and (3) placement of a legend on the document constituting the security which references restrictions on the transferability and sale of the securities.[102]

Offering Exceeding $5 Million The Rule 506 requirements are identical to those of Rule 505 for an offering not exceeding $5 million, with only two exceptions. First, there is no limitation on the size of the issue.[103] Second,

Nonaccredited investors must meet certain qualifications. Specifically, the issuer must reasonably conclude at the time of purchase that each of the Nonaccredited Investors has "such knowledge and experience in financial and business matters that he is capable of evaluating the merits and risks of the prospective investment" (i.e., is a Qualified Investor).[104] In assessing whether a potential investor is a Qualified Investor, the issuer may—under certain circumstances—impute to the investor the knowledge of investor representatives relied upon by the purchaser if such representatives have no conflict of interest and "have such knowledge and experience in financial and business matters that [they] are capable of evaluating . . . the merits and risks of the prospective investment" to the purchaser.[105] Thus, an individual who would not otherwise qualify as a Qualified Investor may be deemed such when the issuer knows he or she is using a Qualified Purchaser or Representative.[106]

Accredited Investors Exception

Section 4(6) of the Securities Act provides that the disclosure provisions of the Act do not apply to the placement of an issue if (1) offers or sales are made solely to "accredited investors," (2) the aggregate offering price of the issue does not exceed $5 million, and (3) there is no "advertising or public solicitation" in connection with the issue.[107] The term "accredited investor" has a similar meaning as in Regulation D.[108]

Private Placement Exception

Section 4(2) of the Securities Act provides that the registration requirements of the Securities Act do not apply to a transaction not involving a public offering of securities.[109] There is no specificity, however, as to precisely what constitutes such an offering. Therefore, issuers typically attempt to comply with Regulation D (described above) so as to be assured of compliance with the Securities Act and use § 4(2) as a fallback. The SEC explicitly states that "an issuer's failure to satisfy all terms and conditions of" Regulation D "shall not raise any presumption that the exemption provided by section 4(2) of the Act is not available."[110]

Regulation A

In the event that neither the intrastate offering exemption nor the Regulation D exemption is available, Regulation A may afford an exemption from the registration requirements of the Securities Act.[111] Regulation A is generally used as a last resort because it involves a number of restrictions and the filing of an offering statement.

The aggregate offering price for the issue cannot exceed $5 million (including no more than $1.5 million offered by all selling security holders).[112] Any sale of securities by the issuer under Regulation A in the 12 months must be applied towards this limit.[113]

Securities may not be offered for sale until an abbreviated offering statement (including a preliminary offering circular) has been filed with the SEC, though the issuer may conduct certain limited activities "to determine whether there is any interest in a contemplated securities offering."[114] Once such a filing is made, the issuer may (1) conduct certain limited public advertising, (2) make oral offers, and (3) make certain written offers through use of a qualified preliminary offering circular.[115] Once the filing is qualified by the SEC, the issuer may also (1) make other written offers so long as they are accompanied by the approved final offering circular, (2) sell the securities so long as the purchaser receives a preliminary or final offering circular at least 48 hours prior to the confirmation of sale to that person.[116]

Unless an affiliate of the issuer cannot resell the securities in the offering, the issuer has had net income from continuing operations in at least one of the two preceding fiscal years.[117]

Registration, Reporting, and Proxy Requirements of the Securities Act and Exchange Act

In the absence of a public offering, the registration, reporting, and proxy solicitation requirements of the Exchange Act will not apply so long as (1) the issuer's securities are not listed on a national securities exchange and (2) no class of securities is held by 500 or more persons of record.[118]

ENDNOTES

1. OIG Advisory Opinion 98-12 at 3; OIG Advisory Opinion 97-5 at 7. See also 56 Fed. Reg. at 35966 ("[W]e believe that a large number of these newly formed entities are designed to have physicians as investors specifically to induce them to use the entity in which they have invested."). The OIG also contends that "the mere opportunity to invest and consequently receive profit distributions" in a nonsafe harbored joint venture may "constitute illegal remuneration" if offered in exchange for or to induce the generation of Federal Program business for the joint venture or fellow investors. OIG Advisory Opinion 97-5 at 10. According to the OIG "[s]uch situations may include arrangements where one or several investors control a sufficiently large stream of referrals to make the venture's financial success highly likely, or where one investor has established a track record with similar ventures or the financial investment is so small that the investors have little or no risk." OIG Advisory Opinion 97-5 at 10.

2. OIG Advisory Opinion 97-5 at 5.

3. Joint Venture Fraud Alert at 65374.

4. Joint Venture Fraud Alert at 65374; OIG Advisory Opinion 98-12 at 3; OIG Advisory Opinion 97-5 at 5, 7.

5. 56 Fed. Reg. at 35068.

6. OIG Advisory Opinion 98-12 at 3; OIG Advisory Opinion 97-5 at 5.

7. See OIG Advisory Opinion 01-17 at 6; OIG Advisory Opinion 97-5 at 6; 56 Fed. Reg. at 35954.

8. 42 C.F.R. § 1001.952(a)(2)(i). Investment interests held by an entity will be deemed to be held by the entity and imputed proportionally to its investors and beyond until all interests are allotted to individuals. 56 Fed. Reg. at 35969.

9. OIG Advisory Opinion 98-12 at 4.

10. 56 Fed. Reg. at 35969.

11. OIG Advisory Opinion 97-5 at 7; Advisory Opinion 01-17 at 7; Advisory Opinion 01-21 at 10; 64 Fed. Reg. at 63537.

12. Compare 64 Fed. Reg. at 63537 (indicating a written stipulation from a joint venture investor will exempt such investor from counting against the 40% ceiling) with OIG Advisory Opinions 03-2, 01-17, and 01-21 (concluding that a hospital does not satisfy the ASC safe harbor requirement that it "not be in a position to make or influence referrals directly or indirectly" when it executes a written stipulation that "significantly constrained" its ability to promote Federal Program business for the ASC joint venture).

13. 64 Fed. Reg. at 63523.

14. 64 Fed. Reg. at 63523.

15. 59 Fed. Reg. at 37204. See also 56 Fed. Reg. at 35967 (defining the difference between "active" and "passive" investors).

16. 59 Fed. Reg. at 37204.

17. 42 C.F.R. § 1001.952(a)(2)(ii).

18. 56 Fed. Reg. at 35968.

19. 42 C.F.R. § 1001.952(a)(4).

20. 42 C.F.R. § 1001.952(a)(4); 56 Fed. Reg. at 35967.

21. 42 C.F.R. § 1001.952(a)(2)(iii).

22. 56 Fed. Reg. at 35968.

23. 42 C.F.R. § 1001.952(a)(2)(iv).

24. 56 Fed. Reg. at 35969.

25. 42 C.F.R. §§ 1001.952(a)(2)(vii).

26. 56 Fed. Reg. at 35970.

27. 56 Fed. Reg. at 35970.

28. 42 C.F.R. § 1001.952(a)(2)(viii).

29. See Chapter 2 for an overview of the additional safe harbor requirements.

30. 64 Fed. Reg. at 63536; OIG Advisory Opinion 98-12 at 5.

31. 64 Fed. Reg. at 63536.

32. 64 Fed. Reg. at 63538.

33. OIG Advisory Opinion 98-12 at 4.

34. 58 Fed. Reg. at 49009; 64 Fed. Reg. at 63536; OIG Advisory Opinion 98-12 at 4 ("There are obvious and legitimate business and professional reasons for surgeons to want to own an ambulatory surgery center in which they personally perform services on a routine basis, [including]. . . personal and patient convenience, professional autonomy, accountability, and quality control."). "In contrast to other investment interest safe harbors which seek to limit investment by individuals in a position to refer, this proposed ASC safe harbor only protects entities whose investment interests are held *entirely* by such individuals." 58 Fed. Reg. at 49009; 64 Fed. Reg. at 63534 (emphasis in original).

35. 42 C.F.R. § 1001.952(r)(4)(viii).

36. OIG Advisory Opinion 97-5 at 7; Advisory Opinion 01-17 at 3, 7; Advisory Opinion 01-21 at 10; 64 Fed. Reg. at 63537.

37. See 64 Fed. Reg. at 63537 (indicating a written stipulation from a joint venture investor will exempt such investor from counting against the 40% ceiling).

38. See OIG Advisory Opinion 01-17 (concluding that a hospital does not satisfy the ASC safe harbor requirement that it "not be in a position to make or influence referrals directly or indirectly" when it executes a written stipulation that "significantly constrained" its ability to promote Federal Program business for the ASC joint venture); OIG Advisory Opinion 01-21 (same); OIG Advisory Opinion 03-2 (same).

39. See OIG Advisory Opinion 01-21 (concluding that there is a "sufficiently low" risk of fraud and abuse in an ASC joint venture where, among other things, the investing hospital agrees in writing that (1) its employed physicians will not refer patients to the ASC or ASC investors, (2) it will not take any action to require or encourage any staff physicians to refer patients to the ASC or ASC investors, (3) it will not track referrals to the ASC or ASC investors, (4) it will not compensate physicians or others based upon the referrals or business they generate for the ASC or ASC investors, and (5) it will inform all staff physicians of the foregoing on an annual basis); OIG Advisory Opinion 01-17 (reaching the same conclusion in an arrangement in which the hospital adopted similar safeguards); OIG Advisory Opinion 03-2 (same). See also OIG Advisory Opinion 97-5 (reaching the same conclusion in analyzing a hospital–physician radiology services joint venture in which the parties did not qualify for the Investment Interests Safe Harbor but adopted similar safeguards to "significantly constrain" the hospital's ability to generate Federal Program business for the joint venture).

40. A person who would typically be deemed to be a Business Source Investor may secure exclusion from such status by (1) executing a written stipulation that he or she will not do so and (2) abiding by such stipulation for the life of his or her investment. 64 Fed. Reg. at 63537.

41. 42 C.F.R. § 1001.952(r)(4) (cross referencing 42 C.F.R. § 1001.952(r)(1)).

42. 42 C.F.R. § 1001.952(r)(4) (cross referencing 42 C.F.R. § 1001.952(r)(2)).

43. 42 C.F.R. § 1001.952(r)(4) (cross referencing 42 C.F.R. § 1001.952(r)(3)). The additional requirement that each physician perform at least one-third of his or her ASC-Approved procedures at the joint venture ASC is designed to minimize the risk of cross-referral arrangements between physicians in separate specialties. 64 Fed. Reg. at 63537. For example, the requirement would prevent safe harbor protection if an orthopedic surgical group and a pain management anesthesia group exchanged interests in each other's respective ASC joint ventures in order to induce referrals across medical specialties.

44. 42 C.F.R. § 1001.952(r)(4)(i).

45. 42 C.F.R. §1001.952(r)(4)(ii). This provision is designed to ensure that the investor's funds are "genuinely at risk" in the joint venture. This provision does not preclude the joint venture from borrowing funds from one or more investors to cover capital or operating expenses. 56 Fed. Reg. at 35970.

46. OIG Advisory Opinion 97-5 at 10. See also 56 Fed. Reg. at 35970.

47. 42 C.F.R. §1001.952(r)(4)(iii).

48. See Chapter 2 for an overview of the additional safe harbor requirements.

49. 56 Fed. Reg. at 35969.

50. OIG Advisory Opinion 97-5 at 7–8, 9.

51. OIG Special Advisory Bulletin on Contractual Joint Ventures (April 2003) ("Joint Venture Advisory Bulletin"); Joint Venture Fraud Alert at 65374.

52. OIG Advisory Opinion 97-5 at 10; Joint Venture Advisory Bulletin; Joint Venture Fraud Alert at 65374.

53. 42 C.F.R. § 1001.952(a)(2)(vii).

54. OIG Advisory Opinion 01-21 at 3 n.2, 9 (determining that sanctions will not be imposed in connection with a physician–hospital joint venture arrangement to establish an ASC even though two of the eight physician investors paid a higher price for investment shares, given that they bought into the joint venture later than the initial six investors and the price differential in the membership interests was equivalent to the fair market value of the appreciation of the value of the membership interests during the intervening period).

55. 64 Fed. Reg. at 63536. "In contrast to other investment interest safe harbors which seek to limit investment by individuals in a position to refer, this proposed ASC safe harbor only protects entities whose investment interests are held *entirely* by such individuals." 58 Fed. Reg. at 49009; 64 Fed. Reg. at 63534 (emphasis in original).

56. OIG Advisory Opinion 01-17 at 7–8.

57. OIG Advisory Opinion 01-17 at 7–8.

58. OIG Advisory Opinion 01-21 at 6; OIG Advisory Opinion 01-17 at 3–4.

59. 42 C.F.R. §1001.952(r)(4)(ii).

60. OIG Advisory Opinion 97-5 at 10.

61. OIG Advisory Opinion 01-21 at 3 n.2, 9 (determining that sanctions will not be imposed in connection with a physician–hospital joint venture arrangement to establish an ASC even though two of the eight physician investors paid a higher price for investment shares, given that they bought into the joint venture later than the initial six investors and the price

differential in the membership interests was equivalent to the fair market value of the appreciation of the value of the membership interests during the intervening period).

62. 42 U.S.C. § 1320a-7(b)(8).

63. DOJ/FTC Health Industry Guidelines § 9(b)(2)(B).

64. Corporate stock is almost invariably deemed to be a security. See *Landreth Timber Co. v. Landreth*, 471 U.S. 681, 692 (1985). So are limited partnership interests. *L&B Hosp. Ventures, Inc. v. Healthcare Int'l*, 894 F.2d 150, 151 (5th Cir. 1990); Carter G. Bishop & Daniel S. Kleinberger, *Limited Liability Companies: Tax and Business Law* (2002) ("Limited Liability Companies") § 11.03[1][c] n.106 (citing cases in which limited partnerships are deemed to be "securities" for purposes of the Securities Act). Although there are credible grounds to contend that LLC membership interests should rarely qualify as a security, the law is sufficiently ambiguous that a joint venture must assume that such interests would be deemed a security. Limited Liability Companies § 11.03[1]. Finally, although general partnership interests are deemed to be exempt from the definition of a security in many contexts, prudence suggests that it must be assumed that such interests might be deemed security interests in a joint venture context. *Williamson v. Tucker*, 645 F.2d 404, 424 (5th Cir. 1981).

65. *Reves v. Ernst & Young*, 494 U.S. 56, 65 (1990).

66. *Reves*, 494 U.S. at 65, 70-71; 15 U.S.C. §§ 77c(a)(3), 78c(3)(a)(10). Commercial paper is typically deemed to be a negotiable note with a maturity date of less than nine months, which is used to fund ongoing operating expenses and is not made available primarily to the general public. Zolman Cavitch, *Business Organizations with Tax Planning*, § 93.03[4] (Mathew Bender 2001). The courts and the SEC also make exception for debt notes structured and distributed in such a way that suggests they need not be regulated in order to protect the investing public. *Reves*, 494 U.S. at 65, 70-71; 15 U.S.C. §§ 77c(a)(3), 78c(3)(a)(10). This exception involves application of a number of amorphous factors, however, and therefore should not be relied upon as a prudent basis for negating registration under the Securities Act. See *Reves*, 494 U.S. at 66-67.

67. 15 U.S.C. § 17l(a).

68. Those issuing securities that qualify for exemption from the registration requirement of the Securities Act may still be held liable for civil penalties, criminal penalties, cease and desist orders, injunctions, and civil damages under the antifraud provisions of the Securities Act and the Exchange Act.

69. 16 U.S.C. § 77(c)(11). Section 3(a)(11) and the associated exemption protect an issue of securities from the registration requirements of §§ 5 and 3(a)(11) of the Securities Act but do not afford protection from the antifraud, civil liability, or other provisions in the Act. 17 C.F.R. § 230.147, Preliminary Note 3.

70. 17 C.F.R. § 230.147, Preliminary Note 1.

71. 17 C.F.R. § 230.147(b)(1). An offer or sale of securities by an issuer shall not be deemed to be part of the same issue as a security if at least six months has passed since the last offer, offer for sale, or sale of the same or similar securities by or for the issuer. 17 C.F.R. § 230.147(b)(2). If the issuer has made an offer or sale in connection with a security within the preceding six months, the SEC will assess the following factors in determining whether the previous offer or sale is "part of the same issue": (1) were the offerings part

of the same plan of financing, (2) do the offerings involve issuance of the same class of securities, (3) are the offerings made at or about the same time, (4) is the same type of consideration to be received, and (5) are the offerings made for the same general purpose. 17 C.F.R. § 230.147, Preliminary Note 3.

72. 17 C.F.R. § 230.147(c).

73. 17 C.F.R. § 230.147(c)(2). The exemption prescribes various timelines to which these calculations apply. 17 C.F.R. § 230.147(c)(2).

74. 17 C.F.R. § 230.147(e).

75. 17 C.F.R. § 230.147(f)(1).

76. 17 C.F.R. § 230.147(f)(1).

77. 17 C.F.R. § 230.147(f)(1).

78. 17 C.F.R. § 230.147(f)(2)-(3).

79. Compliance with any of the three exemptions permits the joint venture to avoid the registration requirements of the Securities Act but does not preclude application of the antifraud, civil liability, or other provisions of federal securities laws. 17 C.F.R. Part 230, Subpart 5, Preliminary Note 1.

80. 17 C.F.R. § 230.504(a). The $1 million threshold includes (1) the securities involved in the issue, and (2) all other securities sold by the joint venture during the 12 months preceding conclusion of the offering at issue. 17 C.F.R. § 230.504(b)(2).

81. This restriction also applies to anyone acting on the issuer's behalf.

82. 17 C.F.R. § 230.504(b)(1). If offers and sales are made in multiple jurisdictions and some subset of the jurisdictions does not require the delivery of the substantive disclosure document, the issuer must nonetheless furnish those solicited in such jurisdictions with a copy of the disclosure document prior to sale. 17 C.F.R. § 230.504(b)(1)(ii).

83. 17 C.F.R. § 230.504(b)(1)(iii).

84. 15 U.S.C. § 77b(a)(15); 17 C.F.R. § 230.501(a).

85. 17 C.F.R. § 230.502(d).

86. 17 C.F.R. § 230.503(d). The SEC recognizes that there may be other methods by which to exercise reasonable care to ensure any transfer or resale of the securities comports with the requirements of or exception to the Securities Act. 17 C.F.R. § 230.503(d).

87. 17 C.F.R. § 230.504(b)(1). If offers and sales are made in multiple jurisdictions and some subset of the jurisdictions does not require the delivery of the substantive disclosure document, the issuer must nonetheless furnish those solicited in such jurisdictions with a copy of the disclosure document prior to sale. 17 C.F.R. § 230.504(b)(1)(ii).

88. 17 C.F.R. § 230.504(b)(1)(iii).

89. 17 C.F.R. §§ 230.505(a), 505(b)(1). The $5 million includes (1) the securities involved in the issue and (2) all other securities sold by the joint venture during the 12 months preceding conclusion of the offering at issue. 17 C.F.R. § 230.505(b)(2)(i).

90. 17 C.F.R. § 230.505(b)(2)(iii).

91. 17 C.F.R. § 230.505(b)(2)(ii).

92. 17 C.F.R. § 230.501(e), cross-referenced in 17 C.F.R. § 230.505(b)(2)(i).

93. 17 C.F.R. § 230.501(e), cross-referenced in 17 C.F.R. § 230.505(b)(2)(i).

94. 17 C.F.R. § 230.501(e), cross-referenced in 17 C.F.R. § 230.505(b)(2)(i).

95. 17 C.F.R. § 230.502(c), cross-referenced in 17 C.F.R. § 230.505(b)(1).

96. 17 C.F.R. § 230.502(b)(1), cross-referenced in 17 C.F.R. § 230.506(b)(1).

97. 17 C.F.R. § 230.502(b)(2), cross-referenced in 17 C.F.R. § 230.506(b)(1).

98. 17 C.F.R. § 230.502(b)(2), cross-referenced in 17 C.F.R. § 230.506(b)(1).

99. 17 C.F.R. § 230.502(b)(1), cross-referenced in 17 C.F.R. § 230.505(b)(1).

100. 17 C.F.R. § 230.502(b)(1), cross-referenced in 17 C.F.R. § 230.505(b)(1).

101. 17 C.F.R. § 230.501(d), cross-referenced in 17 C.F.R. § 230.505(b)(1).

102. 17 C.F.R. § 230.502(d), cross-referenced in 17 C.F.R. § 505(b)(1). The SEC recognizes that there may be other methods by which to exercise reasonable care to ensure any transfer or resale of the securities comports with the requirements of or exception to the Securities Act. 17 C.F.R. § 230.503(d).

103. 17 C.F.R. § 230.506(b).

104. 17 C.F.R. § 230.506(b)(2)(ii).

105. 17 C.F.R. § 230.502(h), cross-referenced in 17 C.F.R. § 230.506(b)(2)(ii).

106. 17 C.F.R. § 230.506(b)(2)(ii).

107. 15 U.S.C. § 77(6). Section 4(6) creates an exemption from the registration requirements of §§ 5 and 3(a)(11) of the Securities Act but does not create an exemption to the antifraud, civil liability, or other provisions in the Act.

108. See note 84 and accompanying text.

109. 15 U.S.C. § 77d(d).

110. 17 C.F.R. Part 230, Subpart 5, Preliminary Note 3.

111. The following companies are excluded from relying upon Regulation A: (1) companies required to file certain reports under the Exchange Act, (2) most foreign issuers, (3) development companies formed with no business purpose or only to merge with other entities, (4) companies issuing certain oil, gas, or mineral rights, and (5) companies subject to certain sanctions involving federal securities laws. 17 C.F.R. § 230.251(a).

112. 17 C.F.R. § 230.251(b).

113. 17 C.F.R. § 230.251(b).

114. 17 C.F.R. §§ 230.251(d)(1), 230.252-230.254.

115. 17 C.F.R. § 230.251(d)(1).

116. 17 C.F.R. § 230.251(d)(2)(i). If a preliminary (rather than a final) circular is delivered prior to the sale, a final circular must be delivered to the purchaser with the confirmation of sale. 17 C.F.R. § 230.251(d)(2)(i).

117. 17 C.F.R. § 230.251(b).

118. See 15 U.S.C. §§ 77, 78l(a) (generally requiring companies issuing securities on a national exchange to register under the Exchange Act) 78l(g)(1) (generally requiring companies to register under the Exchange Act if their securities are held by 500 or more people and certain other requirements are met), 78m(a) (limiting the obligation to publish periodic and other reports to those entities with securities registered under the Exchange Act), 15 U.S.C. § 78o(d) (limiting the obligation to publish similar reports to those entities that have registered securities under the Securities Act).

CHAPTER 8

Structuring the Joint Venture

INTRODUCTION

Hospitals must be mindful of federal regulatory requirements when structuring joint ventures. Such sensitivity is particularly important for tax-exempt hospitals, given that structural considerations can be vital in ensuring that joint venture operations do not threaten the hospital's exempt status or lead to excessive unrelated business income. Structural considerations can also prove central to ensuring compliance with or minimizing burdens under Federal fraud and abuse and federal antitrust laws. This chapter addresses the pertinent compliance concerns in each of the foregoing areas and suggests safeguards through which a joint venture can be structured so as to promote compliance with federal law.

FRAUD AND ABUSE COMPLIANCE

Anti-Kickback

There are no Anti-Kickback Law safe harbor requirements or potential safeguards pertaining to the manner in which the joint venture is structured other than those discussed in connection with selecting investors and operating the joint venture.

Stark Law

Structural Efforts to Avert Implication of the Stark Law

As described in Chapter 2, the Stark Law generally prohibits a physician from referring a Medicare beneficiary requiring DHS to an entity with which the physician has a financial relationship, including a financial relationship that takes the form of an "ownership or investment interest." When a potential investor determines that an investment interest will preclude him or her from referring patients to the joint venture or those compensating the joint venture for items or services, the temptation might arise to attempt to structure the investor's participation in a manner that is indirect and, thereby, ostensibly less likely to implicate the Stark Law referral prohibition.

Given the broad scope of the Stark Law, however, such efforts will not likely be successful. For example, an investor cannot avert the Stark Law by taking bonds or other secured debt (as opposed to equity) in the joint venture because a secured debt holding is deemed to constitute an "ownership or investment interest" implicating the Stark Law.[1] An unsecured debt holding (or convertible security or stock option) in the joint venture also constitutes a financial relationship under the Stark Law.[2] Additionally, a physician will not avert the Stark Law merely by holding his or her ownership investment interest in the joint venture indirectly (e.g., by holding an interest in a juridical entity which, in turn, holds an interest in the joint venture). The Stark Law clearly provides that, under such circumstances, the physician has an ownership interest in the joint venture, thereby implicating the Stark Law, regardless of the number of intervening entities between the physician and joint venture.[3]

Structural Efforts to Ensure Compliance with an Exception to the Stark Law Referral and Billing Prohibition

Nonetheless, structural considerations are imperative when forming a joint venture with physicians to own a hospital or physician practice because the Stark Law exceptions protecting DHS referrals to such entities by physician investors incorporate structural requirements.

Joint Ventures to Own/Operate a Hospital In order to bill for inpatient or outpatient hospital services furnished to Medicare patients referred by an investor-physician, a joint venture hospital must be structured so that the physician's investment interest is in the *entire* hospital and not a constituent department or facility.[4] Thus, investment returns paid to the physician must be derived from the hospital's general net revenues and not from the performance of one or more components of the overall facility. Moreover, the investor must maintain staff privileges at the hospital owned by the joint venture.[5]

Please note that § 507 of P.L. 108-173 makes this exception unavailable until May 18, 2005 for "specialty hospitals" outside of Puerto Rico unless they were in operation or under development as of November 18, 2003 and have not done any of the following since that date: (1) increased the number of physician investors, (2) added certain categories of new clinical services, (3) added bed capacity in contravention of certain restrictions, or (4) violated other requirements to be designated by the Secretary. For purposes of this restriction, a "specialty hospital" is one "primarily or exclusively" engaged in treating patients with a cardiac or orthopedic condition, undergoing surgery, or receiving any other "specialized category of services that the Secretary designates as "inconsistent with the purpose of permitting physician ownership and investment interests in a hospital" under the "Whole Hospital Investment Interest Exception."

Joint Ventures to Own/Operate a Physician Practice In order to bill for DHS furnished to a Medicare beneficiary pursuant to a referral from a physician investor, physician employee, or physician contractor, a joint venture may wish to rely on the Group Practice Exception or the In-Office Ancillary Services Exception. In order to do so, the joint venture must qualify as a "group practice" through compliance with the following structural safeguards:

- The joint venture is a "single legal entity formed primarily for the purpose of being a group practice" and is not organized or owned (in whole or part) by another medical practice and is not part of the hospital.

- The joint venture has at least two physicians as shareholders or employees.

- Each physician shareholder and physician employee uses the joint venture's shared office space, equipment, and personnel to furnish "substantially the full range" of the "patient care services" he or she "routinely performs".

- 75% of the aggregate of all "patient care services" of the joint venture's physician shareholders and physician employees are furnished by the joint venture and billed under the joint venture's billing number.

- The joint venture's overhead and income are distributed according to methods determined before receipt of payment for the services giving rise to such overhead or income.

- The joint venture is a "unified business" with centralized decision-making and utilization review as well as consolidated billing, accounting, and financial reporting.

- Physician shareholders and employees do not receive compensation based on the volume or value of DHS referrals they make other than through qualified productivity bonuses or profit distributions.

- Physician shareholders or employees perform at least 75% of the joint venture's patient-physician encounters.[6]

- Applicable State law permits the entity to qualify as a group practice even though one or more shareholders are not physicians.[7]

TAX COMPLIANCE

When contemplating a joint venture, an exempt hospital must ensure that the arrangement will not jeopardize its exempt status. The appropriate safeguards will vary depending, in substantial part, on how the joint venture is structured.

Use of a Flow-Through Entity

Preserving Exempt Status

When it can do so without jeopardizing its exempt status, an exempt hospital will most often choose to organize a joint venture as a partnership, limited partnership, or limited liability company treated as a partnership for tax purposes (collectively referred to as "Flow-Through Entities").[8] Flow-Through Entities are a preferable vehicle for joint venture arrangements because they pay no tax themselves; rather, they serve as a conduit through which income, losses, and other tax benefits are allotted to investors for taxation at their respective tax rates. Since an exempt hospital generally pays no income tax, it can often retain the entire "pretax" value of the distributions it receives from the joint venture.[9] For-profit partners benefit from such a structure because they avoid double taxation on joint venture proceeds.

The operative question, then, is precisely when and under what circumstances can an exempt hospital participate in a joint venture structured as a Flow-Through Entity without jeopardizing its exempt status. An exempt hospital may serve as a passive investor (i.e., a limited partner or nonmanaging LLC member) in a joint venture structured as a Flow-Through Entity without jeopardizing its exempt status so long as (1) the investment is prudent and (2) the exempt hospital's share of distributed or undistributed revenue from activity "unrelated" to its charitable purpose is not too substantial when compared to its overall charitable activities.[10] When the exempt hospital serves as an active investor (i.e., a general partner or managing LLC member), however, the analysis differs. Under such circumstances, the business activity of the joint venture is imputed directly to the hospital.[11] Therefore, the joint venture will jeopardize the hospital's exemption unless federal courts and the Service determine that the joint venture (1) furthers the hospital's exempt purpose, (2) allows the hospital to operate exclusively for exempt purposes, and (3) is devoid of private inurement or excess private benefit.[12] Each such requirement is addressed below.

The Joint Venture Must Further the Hospital's Charitable Purpose The Service will first inquire whether participation in the joint venture furthers the hospital's exempt purpose.[13] As noted above, the vast majority of nonprofit hospitals are 501(c)(3) "charitable" organizations whose exempt purpose, defined by the "community benefit" standard, is the "promotion of health" for a broad portion of the community.[14] The Service has traditionally been most amenable to finding community benefit (and, therefore, exempt purpose) in joint ventures formed for (1) "creation of a new provider of health care services," (2) "expansion of community health care services," (3) "improvement in treatment modalities," (4) "reduction in health care costs," and (5) "improved patient convenience and access to physicians."[15] The Service has explicitly concluded that joint ventures further a charitable purpose when created to establish or maintain the following facilities for use by a broad section of the community:

- A rehabilitation hospital.[16]

- A psychiatric hospital.[17]

- An acute care hospital.[18]

- A nursing home.[19]

- An outpatient physical therapy clinic.[20]

- An ambulatory surgery center.[21]

- A diagnostic imaging facility.[22]

- A women's health clinic.[23]

- A lithotripsy facility.[24]

- An outpatient dialysis center.[25]

- An outpatient cardiac diagnostic services clinic.[26]

- A home health care agency.[27]

- A medical office building adjacent to the hospital campus in which space is made available to physicians on the hospital staff.[28]

- An elder care facility.[29]

- A cancer treatment center or radiation oncology facility.[30]

- A medical clinic located in an underserved area and treating all patients regardless of ability to pay.[31]

Any such facility must be made available to Medicare and Medicaid beneficiaries.[32]

The Service has also concluded that, although certain components of integrated delivery systems such as physician–hospital organizations ("PHOs") and management services organizations ("MSOs") cannot independently qualify as exempt entities under the community benefit standard, an exempt hospital will not likely jeopardize its charitable status by participating in a PHO or MSO joint venture structured as a Flow-Through Entity so long as the hospital maintains adequate control over the joint venture and prevents private inurement or impermissible private benefit.[33] An exempt hospital will best protect itself by documenting the general cost-savings and clinical benefits associated with the integration arrangement.[34]

The Joint Venture Must Not Impede the Exempt Hospital's Ability to Operate Exclusively For Exempt Purposes Upon establishing that a joint venture generally furthers the exempt hospital's charitable purpose, the Service will inquire whether the joint venture might nonetheless interfere with the hospital's ability to operate exclusively in furtherance of that purpose.[35] Specifically, once it participates in the joint venture, can the hospital still be said to (1) engage "primarily" in activities which meet the community benefit standard or other exempt purpose and (2) ensure that only an insubstantial portion (if any) of its activities are in furtherance of a non-exempt purpose.[36] In making this assessment, federal courts and the Service focus on the "purpose" rather than the "nature" of the hospital's activities. Thus, the mere fact that a hospital engages in a trade or business through a joint venture will not jeopardize its exempt status so long as these activities are undertaken to further its charitable purpose.[37] Nonetheless, if the hospital maintains even a single substantial nonexempt purpose in undertaking the joint venture, it will jeopardize its exemption regardless of the number or importance of exempt purposes.[38] The Service has historically expressed three principal concerns when analyzing whether a hospital's participation in a joint venture will preclude it from operating exclusively for exempt purposes. Those concerns are the protection of exempt assets, the reconciliation of fiduciary duties, and operational control.

Protection of Exempt Assets

The Service will initially scrutinize whether the exempt hospital adequately limits its exposure to financial loss resulting from joint venture activities. The Service has historically been particularly concerned when an exempt hospital acts as a general partner in a joint venture arrangement, contending that its resulting liability under state law for all partnership obligations might interfere with the entity's charitable mission.[39] In such circumstances, the Service inquires whether the exempt hospital has taken prudent steps to "insulate itself" from excessive liability. Principal means of protection previously recognized by the Service include maintenance of adequate insurance by the joint venture, indemnity agreements from other joint venture participants, use of nonrecourse debt on the part of the joint venture, and omission of any guarantee to reimburse limited partners for their losses in connection with the joint venture.[40] The nature of the joint venture's activities will dictate the degree of protection warranted. When structuring a partnership arrangement to limit an exempt hospital's liability for debts resulting from its participation in the joint venture, care should be taken to ensure that such liability restrictions do not subject the partnership to designation as a corporation under § 7701 of the IRC.[41]

Although concerns with exposure of exempt assets will be less pronounced when the exempt hospital serves as a limited partner or LLC member, the Service will heavily scrutinize any contractual pledge by the hospital to assume or guarantee joint venture debts or losses incurred by other joint venture members.[42] Such an arrangement would raise concerns relating to exposure of exempt assets as well as private benefit and private inurement (discussed below). Nonetheless, such an arrangement might be permissible when the guarantee or indemnity is limited in scope and part of a larger commercially reasonable arm's-length transaction.[43]

Reconciliation of Fiduciary Duties

Once the exempt hospital's assets are deemed sufficiently insulated from exposure by the joint venture, both the Service and federal courts will inquire whether the hospital reconciles any fiduciary duties owed to fellow joint venture participants with the hospital's charitable mission. Again, the Service's concern has been most pronounced in instances in which an exempt hospital acts as a general partner in a joint venture arrangement, contending that its resulting fiduciary duty under state law to further the commercial interests of fellow investors might conflict with its charitable mission.[44] The Service recognizes, however, that such a conflict can often be resolved through a legally enforceable agreement among joint venture participants that the exempt hospital's charitable purposes supersede any fiduciary obligation it might otherwise have to maximize the joint venture's profits.[45] To the extent that an exempt hospital incurs such a fiduciary duty under applicable state law when acting as a limited partner or LLC member, the Service would likely require a similar agreement.[46]

Operational Control

Once the joint venture's organizational documents are deemed to provide for the primacy of charitable purposes, the Service will scrutinize whether the exempt hospital is granted sufficient operational control to enforce this requirement. Both the Service and federal courts have indicated that adequate control is most readily secured when the exempt hospital maintains a sufficient majority on the venture's governing board to unilaterally (1) set charges for clinical services, (2) terminate or add clinical services lines, (3) terminate management agreements, and (4) make "fundamental operating decisions."[47] According to the Service, fundamental operating decisions subject to board review should include approval of capital and operating budgets, the timing and amount of distributions, selection of key executives, the acquisition or disposition of health care facilities, execution of contracts exceeding a fixed monetary threshold, changes to service mix, and amendment of the governing documents for the joint venture.[48]

Ensuring adequate operational control on the part of the exempt hospital is more difficult in the absence of its outright majority control over joint venture governance. Throughout the 1980s and early 1990s, the Service approved a number of joint ventures in which charitable purposes were made paramount but the exempt hospital maintained only 50% control (and, in a few cases, less than 50% control).[49] Thereafter, the Service appeared to reverse course, more recently arguing that an exempt hospital's numerical control on a joint venture's governing body is all but necessary to ensure the joint venture is operated to serve charitable purposes.[50] This more stringent position has never been explicitly adopted by federal courts. Indeed, a recent seminal precedent, *Redlands Surgical Services v. Commissioner* suggests that outright majority voting power is not a necessary condition to ensure adequate control on the part of an exempt hospital over a joint venture.[51] Nonetheless, it remains unclear precisely what safeguards must be adopted to ensure sufficient control on the part of the exempt hospital in the absence of majority control on the joint venture board. At present, *Redlands* and *St. David's* provide us with the best guidance as to requirements likely to be imposed by federal courts regardless of whether a joint venture is for clinical services or to form an integrated delivery system.[52]

In *Redlands*, the Ninth Circuit denied exempt status to a nonprofit corporation whose sole function was to serve as co-general partner with a for-profit entity in the operation of a surgical center. With voting control split 50-50 between the two general partners, the Ninth Circuit stated "we look to the binding commitments made between [the nonprofit] and the other parties to ascertain whether other specific powers or rights conferred upon the [nonprofit] might mitigate or compensate for its lack of majority control" and otherwise ensure that the joint venture is operated exclusively for charitable purposes.[53] The court ultimately concluded that no such safeguards existed. Nonetheless, in the course of its analysis, the court suggested (by negative implication) that the following factors might collectively be indicative of formal or informal control:

- Matters on which directors are divided are submitted to binding arbitration before independent arbitrators who are obligated to favor charitable purposes over commercial interests in resolving disputes.

- Where a facility is to be operated under management contract, the contract reserves broad oversight powers to the joint venture, runs for a limited term (perhaps five years or less), is renewable only upon consent of the exempt hospital, permits for-cause termination by the exempt hospital, includes a binding contractual requirement that the management company favor charitable purposes over profits, and calculates compensation for the management company in a manner that provides no disincentive to charity care (e.g., a flat fee payment or a percentage-of-revenue payment that explicitly includes charity care as revenue).[54]

- Where a medical advisory group is used, the group is composed of physicians with no economic interest in the joint venture.[55]

- The exempt hospital reserves the right to implement a quality assurance program for medical care at any facility operated by the joint venture.[56]

- The facility operated by the joint venture furnishes substantial charity care and maintains a substantial Medicaid utilization level.[57]

The subsequent ruling by the Fifth Circuit in *St. David's Health Care System v. United States*, however, adds further confusion as to what—if any—safeguards can be adopted to ensure adequate control by a nonprofit member of a joint venture in the absence of a voting majority on the joint venture's governing body. In *St. David's*, a nonprofit entity contributed its hospital facility to a joint venture with a for profit entity, and the joint venture was managed by a company affiliated with the for-profit partner. The Service concluded that St. David's lacked requisite control over the joint venture to ensure operation exclusively for charitable purposes, and therefore revoked the System's exempt status. Although, control of the joint venture's governing body was split 50-50 between the parties, the joint venture's governing documents included a number a safeguards to protect St. David's charitable mission. Safeguards included:

- A mandate in the partnership agreement requiring that partnership facilities be operated in accordance with the community benefit standard (including acceptance of Medicare and Medicaid patients, treating patients with emergency conditions without regard to ability to pay, maintaining an open medical staff, providing public health programs of educational benefit to the community, and providing "quality health care at a reasonable cost" to the community).

- St. David's explicit right to terminate unilaterally the management agreement if the management company takes any action with a "material probability of adversely affecting" St. David's exempt status.

- Provision that no measure can pass the partnership board without support from a majority of the board members appointed by St. David's.

- St. David's explicit right to appoint the initial CEO for the partnership, subject to the veto of the for-profit partner.

- The explicit right of either St. David's or the for-profit partner to unilaterally remove the CEO.

- St. David's explicit right to initiate dissolution of the partnership if it receives legal advice from an attorney acceptable to both joint venture partners that continued participation in the partnership will hinder St. David's tax-exempt status.[58]

In light of the foregoing safeguards, the trial court had awarded summary judgment to St. David's, ruling that—as a matter of law—St. David's exercised requisite control over the joint venture. However, the Fifth Circuit reversed the trial court decision, ruling that—notwithstanding all of the safeguards enumerated above—there was a jury question as to whether St. David's had ceded such control over the joint venture to its for-profit partner that St. David's was no longer operated exclusively for charitable purposes. In so ruling, the Fifth Circuit questioned whether the above-referenced safeguards would provide St. David's with sufficient effective control over operation of the joint venture to ensure exclusive operation for charitable purposes absent majority voting control. Specifically the Court made the following findings:

- With control of only 50% of the partnership's governing board, St. David's can only "veto"—rather than "initiate"—action through the joint venture in furtherance of St. David's charitable goals.

- The partnership's hospital would be managed—through a long-term contract—by a for-profit management company affiliated with the for-profit joint venture partner and compensated based upon partnership revenues.[59]

- The management agreement might not permit sufficient oversight by the partnership over the daily operation of the partnership's facilities.

- The principal means available to St. David's to ensure supremacy of charitable interests (i.e., termination of the management agreement, litigation with the management company, termination of the CEO, or dissolution of the partnership) were extraordinary steps which might not be taken in response to daily operational concerns involving charitable interests.

Given the recent rulings in *Redlands* and *St. David's*, there is substantial ambiguity as to what safeguards would, in the absence of 51% majority voting control, be deemed sufficient to permit an exempt hospital to ensure that a joint venture in which it participates is operated exclusively in furtherance of the hospital's charitable purposes. Thus, pending further guidance from federal courts or the Service exempt, hospitals participating in such ventures—at least those structured as flow-through entities—might deem it advisable to insist on 51% voting control on the governing board and in connection with all major governance decisions. Management contracts for joint venture facilities should also be of limited duration and provide for reasonable oversight of the daily operations of the joint venture.

Private Inurement or Impermissible Private Benefit An exempt hospital is prohibited from conveying private inurement or impermissible private benefit. Violation of either prohibition will result in loss or denial of exempt status.[60] The "mere fact" that an exempt hospital enters into a joint venture with private parties who receive a return on their capital investment does not establish that the exempt hospital has impermissibly conferred private benefit."[61] Nonetheless, the Service has taken the position that any private benefit furnished by the exempt hospital or the joint venture itself must be "qualitatively incidental" (i.e., be a "necessary concomitant of the activity that benefits the public at large") and "quantitatively incidental" (i.e., be "insubstantial when viewed in relationship to the public benefit conferred by the activity.").[62] Moreover, pursuant to the private inurement restriction, remuneration may be furnished by the exempt hospital or the joint venture itself to one of the exempt hospital's "insiders" only as part of a commercially reasonable exchange (i.e., an exchange involving terms and payments equivalent to transactions negotiated at arm's length).[63] As noted above, one commentator has defined the term "insider" to include any person who "has the ability to control or otherwise influence the actions of the tax-exempt organization so as to cause the benefit."[64] On occasion, the Service has suggested that control over a discrete segment of an exempt organization may result in an individual's classification as an insider. As further noted above, the Service has conceded that a physician does not become an "insider" at an exempt hospital merely by securing staff privileges at the facility.[65]

In general the Service and federal courts have closely scrutinized the following factors in determining whether a joint venture gives rise to private inurement or impermissible private benefit:

Factors Helpful to a Positive Decision

- Profits and losses are allocated between the joint venture partners or members according to their respective equity interests which, in turn, are proportionate to their respective capital contributions.[66]

- Any financing, assets, guarantees, or services provided by the exempt hospital to the joint venture are furnished at market rates.[67]

- The compensation and other terms in any management contract involving the joint venture are commercially reasonable (i.e., similar to those in similar agreements negotiated at arm's-length).[68]

- The joint venture receives fair market value compensation for all items, services, or payments it provides to investors or third parties.[69]

- The exempt hospital receives dissolution distributions equivalent to its capital account balance and equity stake.[70]

- The exempt hospital receives the right to purchase any equipment or facility owned by the joint venture upon termination.[71]

- Any new facility or integrated delivery system created by the joint venture maintains an open medical staff.[72]

- Debt assumed by the exempt hospital upon entry into a pre-existing joint venture is collateralized, non-recourse debt.[73]

Factors Harmful to a Positive Decision

- "[T]here is a disproportionate allocation of profits and losses to the nonexempt" joint venture participants.[74]

- The exempt hospital makes loans to the joint venture that are "commercially unreasonable" due to a low interest rate, inadequate security, or other commercially unreasonable terms.[75]

- The exempt hospital provides property or services to the joint venture at less than fair market value or pursuant to terms that are not commercially reasonable.[76]

- The joint venture provides goods or services to nonexempt investors or third parties at less than fair market value.[77]

- Risk asymmetry (i.e., the exempt hospital incurs a disproportionately large portion of the joint venture's downside risk or receives a disproportionately limited portion of the joint venture's upside potential).[78]

- Any new facility or integrated delivery system created by the joint venture will be available only to select members of the exempt hospital's medical staff.[79]

- A facility owned by the joint venture is operated under a management contract for an extended term, renewable thereafter at the sole discretion of the management company.[80]

- The exempt hospital executes a covenant not to compete with the joint venture or other ventures sponsored by the non-exempt joint venture participants.[81]

The Service has identified one category of transactions which, in its opinion, results *per se* private inurement. Specifically, the sale of a gross or net revenue stream in a hospital department to a joint venture comprised in part of staff physicians will likely constitute private inurement thereby jeopardizing the hospital's exempt status.[82]

Summary Collectively, the Service and federal courts have provided guidance as to when a joint venture will be deemed to further a charitable purpose, the requisite safeguards that must be adopted to protect the exempt hospital's assets, the necessary protections to ensure that the exempt hospital's fiduciary duties to joint venture participants do not interfere with its charitable mission, and the circumstances under which joint venture activity might result in inurement or impermissible private benefit. Substantial ambiguity remains, however, in identifying the precise safeguards necessary to ensure that an exempt hospital maintains requisite control over joint venture activities in the absence of majority representation on the venture's governing board. *Redlands* and *St. David's* currently provide the most pertinent guidance. In determining the array of appropriate safeguards to ensure sufficient control by the exempt hospital under such circumstances, one must be particularly cautious in connection with disposition arrangements (i.e., arrangements such as a whole-hospital joint venture in which the exempt hospital has pledged all of its assets to the joint venture). The Service would seemingly be more likely to seek revocation of a hospital's exempt status for lack of control over such a joint venture rather than an ancillary services arrangement in which the exempt hospital retains substantial assets and continues furnishing services in its own right in compliance with the community benefit standard.[83]

Minimizing Unrelated Business Income

Notwithstanding its general exemption from federal income tax liability, an exempt hospital will, nonetheless, be taxed at corporate rates on the modified gross income it receives in connection with any "trade or business" that it "regularly carries on" and which is "not substantially related to" its exempt mission.[84] Moreover, excessive unrelated business income could ultimately jeopardize its exempt status. Therefore, exempt hospitals should structure their joint venture activities so as to minimize the unrelated business income attributable to them.

As noted above, to the extent it can do so without jeopardizing its exempt status, a hospital and its joint venture partners will most often choose to organize a joint venture as a Flow-Through Entity so as to avoid taxation at the joint venture level. The operative question, then, is under what circumstances will an exempt hospital incur unrelated business income tax liability for participating in a joint venture structured in this manner. The answer is as follows: The exempt hospital will incur tax liability on its share of all modified gross income generated by the Flow-Through Entity joint venture from any "trade or business" in which the joint venture is "regularly engaged" and which is "not substantially related to" the hospital's exempt purpose. The hospital will incur this liability irrespective of whether the unrelated income has been distributed to it by the joint venture.[85] If the amount of unrelated business income attributable to the hospital becomes too great, its exempt status will be jeopardized.

The overwhelming majority of hospital-sponsored joint venture arrangements involve the conduct of a trade or business on a regular basis. Thus, the determination as to whether such trade or business is "substantially related" to the hospital's exempt purpose will dictate whether the income is subject to taxation.[86] In order to be substantially related, the joint venture's business or trade activities must have a substantial "causal relationship" with or "contribute importantly" to the hospital's exempt purpose (e.g., furnishing of care to a broad portion of the community).[87] In making this determination, the Service is mindful as to whether the "size and extent" of the trade or business activities are "larger" than "reasonably necessary" for the performance of the hospital's exempt functions.[88] If so, that excess will generate gross income potentially subject to taxation.[89]

Federal statute explicitly provides that any trade or business carried on by an exempt hospital for the convenience of its members, students, patients, officers, or employees must be considered to be substantially related to the hospital's exempt purposes.[90] The term "patient" is defined to include (1) hospital inpatients, (2) hospital outpatients, (3) individuals referred for specific diagnostic or treatment procedures furnished by hospital-affiliated personnel at a hospital facility, (4) residents of a hospital-affiliated extended care facility, (5) those receiving follow-up or pre-admission radiology or laboratory testing, and (6) individuals receiving medical service in their residence in a hospital-administered home care program.[91] The Service has applied the carve-out to conclude that such activities as operation of an on-site parking facility, cafeteria, or coffee shop for use by hospital patients, visitors, and staff will not generate unrelated business income.[92]

Absent application of the foregoing statutory exception, the Service will apply a facts-and-circumstances test to assess whether joint venture activity is substantially related to the hospital's exempt mission. In doing so, the Service will view favorably any indication that the activity involves the "laying of hands" on a patient for clinical treatment.[93] The Service has applied this standard in concluding that income from the following activities will not generate unrelated business income:

- Joint venture to establish and operate an ambulatory surgery center.[94]
- Joint venture to establish and operate a diagnostic imaging center.[95]
- Joint venture to establish a radiation therapy center.[96]
- Joint venture to establish and operate a long-term care nursing home.[97]
- Joint venture to establish an elder care facility.[98]
- Joint venture to establish and operate a freestanding women's health center.[99]
- Joint venture to operate an acute care hospital.[100]
- Joint venture to establish and operate an acute care hospital.[101]
- Joint venture to establish and operate a psychiatric hospital.[102]
- Joint venture to operate a rehabilitation hospital.[103]
- Joint venture to establish and operate a rehabilitation hospital.[104]
- Joint venture to renovate and operate an outpatient rehabilitation clinic.[105]
- Joint venture to establish and operate a cardiac diagnostic services facility.[106]
- Joint venture to establish and operate a home health agency.[107]
- Joint venture to establish and operate an outpatient dialysis facility.[108]
- Joint venture to establish a joint operating company to provide management and oversight of hospitals integrated through a virtual merger.[109]
- Joint venture among several proximate exempt hospitals to furnish clinical laboratory services to their respective inpatients and outpatients (but *not* to nonpatients).[110]

It should be noted that the Service has concluded that revenues from a MSO joint venture will not be deemed "substantially" related to an exempt hospital's charitable mission and will therefore generate unrelated business income tax.[111] Revenues derived from a PHO joint venture's services to physicians in private practice are also deemed not to be "substantially" related to an exempt hospital's charitable mission and will therefore generate unrelated business income tax.[112] Revenues derived from PHO services to the exempt hospital and its patients, however, will not give rise to unrelated business income tax because they are deemed to qualify for the statutory exemption described above.[113]

Once an exempt hospital's gross income from unrelated joint venture business activities is identified, pretax deductions and modifications are made. As noted above, permissible deductions generally consist of the following offsets to unrelated business taxable income: (1) a $1,000 "specific deduction," (2) deductible business expenses "directly connected" with the conduct of the business activity generating the unrelated business income, and (3) charitable contributions equivalent to 10% of unrelated business income if such deduction were not made.[114] The net operating loss deduction provided by IRC § 172 is allowed as an offset to unrelated business taxable income.[115] The net operating loss carryover, however, shall be determined without taking into account the "specific deduction" or any income or deduction that is not included under § 511 in computing unrelated business taxable income.[116] Once these deductions are made, numerous additional modifications can be made to further reduce taxable income. These modifications are described in detail in Chapter 3.

Use of a Non-Flow-Through Entity

Preserving Exempt Status

When there is substantial doubt or ambiguity as to whether a joint venture will further an exempt hospital's charitable purpose or doubt as to whether it can be structured so as to ensure the requisite degree of control on the part of the exempt hospital, the hospital may consider creation of a taxable corporate subsidiary, in the form of a C corporation or a limited liability company taxable as a corporation, to participate in the venture.[117] So long as the subsidiary is incorporated and operated for a legitimate business purpose, is treated as a separate legal entity (i.e., corporate formalities are observed such as separate accounts, separate personnel, distinct facilities, and no majority overlap of officers and directors), and is not used by the exempt hospital as a conduit for indirect private inurement, the subsidiary's activities should pose no risk to the parent's exempt status.[118] Moreover, use of such a subsidiary affords greater protection to the exempt hospital than a Flow-Through Entity with respect to financial, civil, and criminal liability for the acts of the joint venture. Furthermore, the subsidiary will have access to capital through the equity market as well as greater operational flexibility than an exempt entity. Finally, post-tax dividend distributions to the exempt hospital will not give rise to unrelated business income liability.[119]

Likewise, where the activities involve a substantial portion of the exempt hospital's assets or activities, it may wish to secure a private letter ruling.

Minimizing Unrelated Business Income

Notwithstanding its general exemption from federal income tax liability, an exempt hospital will, nonetheless, be taxed at corporate rates on the modified gross income it receives in connection with any "trade or business" that it "regularly carries on" and that is "unrelated to" its exempt mission.[120] Moreover, excessive unrelated business income could ultimately jeopardize its exempt status. Therefore, exempt hospitals should structure their joint venture activities so as to minimize the unrelated business income attributable to them.

If a joint venture will be regularly engaged in a trade or business unrelated to the exempt hospital's charitable purpose, the hospital should give strong consideration to structuring the joint venture as a C corporation or LLC taxed as a corporation. Although the joint venture's activities will be taxed at the subsidiary level, neither income received by nor distributions paid by the subsidiary will generate unrelated business income for the hospital.[121] One caveat, however, is worth noting. Interest, annuities, royalties, and rents received by the exempt hospital from the subsidiary and unrelated to the hospital's exempt purpose will generate unrelated business income if the hospital maintains 50% or greater control over the subsidiary.[122] This requirement is enforced even where the income derives from an unrelated activity that is not "regularly carried on" by the exempt hospital or the joint venture subsidiary.[123]

ANTITRUST COMPLIANCE

The principal antitrust concern associated with structuring a joint venture is exemption from making a HSR filing. If the joint venture is formed as a partnership or limited partnership, no HSR filing will be required.[124] Formation of a joint venture in the form of an LLC will similarly not necessitate an HSR filing unless two or more separately controlled businesses are contributed to the LLC upon formation and at least one party retains a 50% or greater interest in the joint venture.[125] Finally, formation of a joint venture in the form of a corporation (or an LLC involving the contribution of two or more businesses under the 50% control of at least one party), will necessitate an HSR filing only if:

- The capital and credit extended by joint venture participants to the joint venture exceeds $200 million.

- The capital and credit extended by joint venture participants to the joint venture exceeds $50 million and either:

  - The joint venture will have $100 million or more in assets and two or more joint venture investors maintain $10 million in assets or annual net sales; or

  - The joint venture will have $10 million or more in assets, one of the investors maintains $10 million in assets or annual net sales, and a second investor maintains $100 million or more in net sales or total assets.[126]

SECURITIES COMPLIANCE

As noted in Chapter 5, issuance of a financial instrument will only be regulated under the Securities Act or Exchange Act if the instrument qualifies as a "security" under federal law. Thus, those forming a joint venture might be tempted to structure it in a manner so that equity interests in the venture are less likely to be deemed a security (e.g., choose a general partnership form over that of a corporation or limited partnership).[127] This is an infeasible strategy. The term "security" is interpreted with such breadth by the SEC and federal courts that the venture should assume that any corporate stock, limited partnership, and limited liability company membership interests would be so designated under the Act. Efforts to comply with federal securities laws should focus on invoking an appropriate exemption from the registration requirements of the Securities Act and securing derivative protection from the Exchange Act registration and reporting requirements.

ENDNOTES

1. 42 C.F.R. § 411.354(b)(1); 66 Fed. Reg. at 870–871.

2. 42 C.F.R. § 411.354(c); 66 Fed. Reg. at 870.

3. 42 C.F.R. § 411.354(b)(5).

4. 42 U.S.C. § 1395nn(d)(3); 42 C.F.R. § 411.356(c)(3). If the hospital is located in Puerto Rico, however, the physician's investment interest may be in a subdivision or department of the facility. 42 U.S.C. § 1395nn(d)(1); 42 C.F.R. § 411.356(c)(2).

5. 42 U.S.C. § 1395nn(d)(3); 42 C.F.R. § 411.356(c)(3). If the hospital is located in Puerto Rico, however, the Investing Physician need not have privileges there in order to make Medicare DHS referrals to the institution. 42 U.S.C. § 1395nn(d)(1); 42 C.F.R. § 411.356(c)(2).

6. 42 U.S.C. § 1395nn(h)(4); 42 C.F.R. § 411.352. See also 66 Fed. Reg. at 899 (addressing ownership of a group practice by nonphysician investors).

7. 66 Fed. Reg. 899.

8. In fact, when two parties cooperate on an ongoing basis for mutual profit, the Service and federal courts may conclude that, as a matter of law, a partnership results for tax purposes (even if formation of a partnership is contrary to the parties' intent or desire). See, for example, *Commissioner v. Culbertson*, 337 U.S. 733, 742 (1949).

9. An exception to this general rule arises when joint venture activity results in the generation of unrelated business income. See the section in this chapter about minimizing unrelated business income.

10. Michael I. Sanders, *Joint Ventures Involving Tax-Exempt Organizations* (2nd ed. 2000) ("Sanders") § 4.3. See Internal Revenue Code ("IRC") §§ 513(a), 511(a)(1); 26 C.F.R. ("Treas. Reg.") §§ 1.511-1, 1.513(a)(1). See also the later section in this chapter for a discussion of unrelated business income. There is some ambiguity as to the conditions under which the Service will deem an LLC member to be "passive" for purposes of this standard. Sanders § 4.3. Therefore, special care should be taken when relying on this provision to ensure that the exempt hospital's powers as an LLC member are sufficiently circumscribed so that it is clearly a "passive" participant in the joint venture.

11. IRS § 512(c); Rev. Rul. 98-15 (March 4, 1998) (citing *Butler v. Commissioner*, 36 T.C. 1097 (1961)); *Ward v. Commissioner*, 20 T.C. 332, 343-344 (1953), *aff'd*, 224 F.2d 547 (9th Cir. 1955).

12. See, for example, *Plumstead Theatre Society v. Commissioner*, 74 T.C. 1324, 1333-1334 (1980) (ruling that exempt organization's participation as a general partner in a limited partnership joint venture did not result in loss of exempt status where the limited partnership was operated to further a charitable purpose, the limited partners received no control over the joint venture's activities, and no private benefit or private inurement resulted from the arrangement), *aff'd* 675 F.2d 244, 244-245 (9th Cir. 1982); Rev. Rul. 98-15 (March 4, 1998) ("A 501(c)(3) organization may form and participate in a partnership, including an LLC treated as a partnership for federal income tax purposes, and meet the operational test if participation in the partnership furthers a charitable purpose and the partnership arrangement permits the exempt organization to act exclusively in furtherance of its exempt purpose and only incidentally for the benefit of the for-profit partners.").

13. Rev. Rul. 98-15 (March 4, 1998); PLR 9616005 (Dec. 19, 1995); PLR 9345057 (Aug. 20, 1993); GCM 39862 (Nov. 21, 1991); PLR 9105029 (Nov. 6, 1990); PLR 9105031 (Nov. 6, 1990); PLR 9021050 (Feb. 26, 1990); PLR 8925052 (March 28, 1989); GCM 39732 (Nov. 4, 1987); GCM 39005 (June 28, 1983).

14. *Redlands Surgical Services v. Commissioner*, 113 T.C. 47, 73 ("The promotion of health for the benefit of the community is a charitable purpose" so long as the provider serves a "sufficiently large and indefinite class."), *aff'd* 242 F.3d 904 (9th Cir. 2001); Rev. Rule 83-157 (Jan. 1, 1983); Rev. Rul. 69-545.

15. PLR 9352030 (Oct. 8, 1993). See also GCM 39732 (Nov. 4, 1987) (finding that a series of joint ventures each serves a charitable purpose when established to "provide better medical services to the public" through the establishment of new clinical services or new

clinical facilities); GCM 39862 (Nov. 21, 1991) ("We recognize that there may well be legitimate purposes for joint ventures, whether analyzed under the Anti-Kickback Law or the Tax Code. These may include raising needed capital; bringing new services or a new provider to a hospital's community; sharing the risk inherent in a new activity; or pooling diverse areas of expertise.").

16. PLR 9323030 (March 16, 1993); PLR 9319044 (Feb. 18, 1993); PLR 9035072 (June 7, 1990).

17. PLR 8903060 (Oct. 25, 1988); PLR 8432014 (April 9, 1984).

18. PLR 9319044 (Feb. 18, 1993); PLR 9308034 (Nov. 30, 1992); PLR 9204048 (Oct. 30, 1991).

19. PLR 8717057 (Jan. 28, 1987).

20. GCM 39732 (Nov. 4, 1987).

21. GCM 39732 (Nov. 4, 1987); PLR 8817039 (Jan. 29, 1988); PLR 8946067 (Aug. 24, 1989); PLR 8941006 (June 29, 1989); PLR 9345057 (Aug. 20, 1993); PLR 9407022 (Nov. 22, 1993); PLR 9709014 (Nov. 26, 1996); PLR 8638131 (June 30, 1986); PLR 8709051 (Dec. 3, 1986); PLR 8936077 (June 19, 1989); PLR 8931083 (May 15, 1989); PLR 88806057 (Nov. 17, 1987); PLR 8807012 (Oct. 28, 1987), PLR 8715039 (Jan. 13, 1987); PLR 85311069 (May 10, 1985).

22. PLR 9122061 (March 6, 1991); PLR 9105029 (Nov. 6, 1990); PLR 9024085 (March 22, 1990); PLR 9021050 (Feb. 26, 1990); PLR 8833038 (May 20, 1988); PLR 8833009 (May 19, 1988); GCM 39732 (Nov. 4, 1987); PLR 8631094 (May 7, 1986); PLR 8621059 (Feb. 25, 1986); PLR 8344099 (Aug. 5, 1983); PLR 8206093 (Nov. 10, 1981).

23. PLR 8727080 (April 10, 1987).

24. PLR 8936047 (June 13, 1989).

25. PLR 9645018 (Aug. 9, 1996); PLR 9637050 (June 18, 1996); PLR 8705089 (Nov. 7, 1986).

26. PLR 8909036 (Dec. 7, 1988).

27. PLR 8945063 (Aug. 17, 1989); PLR 8943050 (July 31, 1989); PLR 8534089 (May 31, 1985).

28. Rev. Rul. 69-464; PLR 9739041 (June 30, 1997); PLR 8940039 (July 10, 1989); PLR 8506102 (Nov. 16, 1984); PLR 8312129 (Dec. 23, 1982); PLR 8301003 (Oct. 15, 1982).

29. PLR 9518014 (Feb. 1, 1995).

30. PLR 8925052 (March 28, 1989); PLR 8915065 (Jan. 23, 1989).

31. PLR 8616005 (Dec. 19, 1995).

32. Rev. Rul. 98-15; Rev. Rul. 69-545. See also, for example, PLR 9352030 (Oct. 8, 1993) (ruling that a hospital's efforts to expand and renovate its rehabilitative care facilities through a joint venture with a for-profit entity would not undermine its exempt status where, among other things, the partnership facility will continue to treat patients regardless of their ability to pay and will accept Medicare and Medicaid patients); PLR 9518014 (Feb. 1, 1995) (affirming that a nonprofit hospital's joint venture with a for-profit entity to furnish elder care services furthers an exempt purpose where, among other things, 4 of the 54 resident beds would be reserved for financially needy patients who will pay a reduced rate); PLR 9021050 (Feb. 26, 1990) (affirming that a hospital's joint venture with a for-profit entity to furnish elder care services furthers an exempt purpose where the joint venture facility would "be open the public and operated on a non-discriminatory basis."). See also PLR 39862 (Nov. 21, 1991) ("Nearly every hospital that is an exempt organization described in section 501(c)(3) participates in the Medicare and Medicaid programs. In the usual case, doing so is a virtual requirement for exemption.").

33. FY95 CPE Text at 155-158; Unpublished PLR to Williamsburg Community Hospital (Sept. 29, 1994) ("Williamsburg Ruling"), reprinted in EOTR 1323 (Dec. 1994).

34. See FY95 CPE Text at 156 (listing "factors to consider" in determining whether an exempt hospital jeopardizes its exempt status by participation in a PHO).

35. *St. David's Health Care System v. United States*, 2003 U.S. App. Lexis 22851 at *6–*7 (5th Cir.); *Redlands Surgical Services*, 113 TC at 75, 77–86; *Plumstead*, 74 TC at 1333–1334; Rev. Rul. 98-15 (March 4, 1998); PLR 9645018 (Aug. 9, 1996); PLR 9616005 (Dec. 19, 1995); PLR 9345057 (Aug. 20, 1993); PLR 9308034 (Nov. 30, 1992); GCM 39862 (Nov. 21, 1991); PLR 9105029 (Nov. 6, 1990); PLR 9021050 (Feb. 26, 1990); PLR 8925052 (March 28, 1989); GCM 39732 (Nov. 4, 1987); GCM 39005 (June 28, 1983).

36. Treas. Reg. § 1.501(c)(3)-1(c)(1).

37. *Est of Hawaii v. Commissioner*, 71 T.C. 1067, 1079 (1979) (citation omitted). See also Treas. Reg. § 1.501(c)(3)-1(e) ("An organization may meet the requirements of section 501(c)(3) although it operates a trade or business as a substantial part of its activities, if the operation of such trade or business is in furtherance of the organization's exempt purpose or purposes and if the organization is not organized and operated for the primary purpose of carrying on an unrelated trade or business.").

38. *Redlands Surgical Services*, 113 T.C. at 71–72; *American Campaign Academy*, 92 T.C. 1053, 1065 (1989). See also *Better Business Bureau of Washington, D.C. v. United States*, 326 U.S. 279, 283 (1945); *Housing Pioneers* 65 T.C. TCM 2191 (denying tax exempt status to a general partner in a partnership providing low-income housing when a substantial purpose of the activity was to benefit commercial interests of for profit partners), *aff'd* 58 F.3d 401 (9th Cir. 1995).

39. GCM 39005 (June 28, 1993) ("Notwithstanding an established charitable purpose, however, conflicts with charitable goals can nevertheless arise in a limited partnership situation because certain statutory obligations are imposed upon a general partner" such as "assumption of all liabilities by the general partner."); GCM 39862 (Nov. 21, 1991) ("Hospital participation in a joint venture is inconsistent with exemption, then, if . . . there is inadequate protection against financial loss by the hospital."); PLR 8638131 (June 30, 1986) (concluding that a joint venture arrangement with for-profit participants would not affect an exempt participant's exempt status where provisions in the joint venture documents resulted in "the protection of exempt assets against loss.").

40. PLR 9709014 (Nov. 26, 1996); PLR 9345057 (Aug. 20, 1993); PLR 9323030 (March 16, 1993); PLR 9319044 (Feb. 18, 1993); PLR 9308034 (Nov. 30, 1992); PLR 9122061 (March 6, 1991); PLR 9035072 (June 7, 1990); PLR 8945063 (Aug. 17, 1989); PLR 8943050 (July 31, 1989); PLR 8909036 (Dec. 7, 1988); PLR 8727080 (April 10, 1987) (tax-exempt general partner protected by insurance and indemnity agreement); PLR 8638131 (June 30, 1986) (concluding that a joint venture arrangement with for-profit participants would not affect an exempt participant's exempt status where provisions in the joint venture documents resulted in "the protection of exempt assets against loss."). See also *Plumstead Theatre Society*, 74 T.C. at 1333-1334 (Ruling that a tax exempt entity's participation as a general partner in a limited partnership advancing charitable purposes would not result in the loss of exempt status where, among other things, "[p]etitioner is not obligated for the return of any capital contribution made by the limited partners from its own funds.").

41. See Treas. Reg. § 301.7701-2 (providing that a partnership may be deemed a corporation for tax purposes if it evinces more than two of the following characteristics: centralized

management, continuity of life, free transferability of interests, and limited liability); GCM 39546 (Aug. 15, 1986); PLR 8506102 (Nov. 16, 1984).

42. GCM 39862 (Nov. 21, 1991) (rejecting a joint venture in which the partnership agreement made the exempt hospital liable for any losses incurred by limited partners and required the exempt hospital to establish a "loss reserve" for such contingency); PLR 9616005 (Dec. 19, 1995) (approving exempt organization's participation in a general partnership with a for-profit entity where the exempt organization does not guarantee the venture's debt and may not borrow additional funds without the exempt entity's consent); PLR 9345057 (Aug. 20, 1993) (approving a joint venture and emphasizing that the exempt organization "is in no way obligated for the return of any capital contributions to the limited partners."); PLR 9352030 (Oct. 8, 1993) (affirming that an exempt hospital's participation in a joint venture with for-profit entities would not affect its tax-exempt status where, among other things, the hospital is "not required to place any" of its assets at risk other than those directly contributed to the joint venture).

43. PLR 8915065 (Jan. 23, 1989) (approving exempt entity's participation in a joint venture where the exempt entity guarantees certain joint venture debts because the guarantee was secured by sufficient collateral and required repayment at a premium); PLR 8506102 (Nov. 16, 1984) (approving a joint venture where the exempt entity guarantees a loan made to the joint venture because financial liability under the guarantee is limited in amount and required by a third-party lender, and payments made under the guarantee are subject to commercially reasonable interest backed by collateral from the limited partners).

44. GCM 39005 (June 28, 1993); GCM 39862 (Nov. 21, 1991).

45. For example, PLR 9345057 (Aug. 20, 1993); PLR 8936077 (June 19, 1989); PLR 9345057 (Aug. 20, 1993); PLR 9352030 (Oct. 8, 1993); PLR 8945063 (Aug. 17, 1989); PLR 9308034 (Nov. 30,1992). The law in some states may preclude such a provision in favor of fiduciary protections to investors, thereby necessitating that the joint venture be organized in a different state. Sanders at 137.

46. Rev. Rul. 98-15 (March 4, 1998).

47. *Redlands Surgical Services*, 113 T.C. at 79–80; Rev. Rul. 98-15 (March 4, 1998). See also, for example, PLR 9637050 (June 18, 1996) (exempt organization's participation in a joint venture with a for-profit partner will not affect its exempt status given that the exempt organization "will retain majority ownership and control of" the joint venture, including its operational "policies and guidelines," to ensure that charitable purposes prevail when in conflict with business concerns); PLR 9709014 (Nov. 26, 1996) (exempt organization's participation in a joint venture with a for-profit partner will not affect its exempt status given that "management and control" of the joint venture "rests exclusively" with the exempt organization "as the sole general partner."); PLR 8638131 (June 30, 1986) (exempt organization's participation in a joint venture with a for-profit partner will not affect its exempt status given that the exempt entity has "effective control" of the joint venture "through its 60% general partnership interest."); PLR 8936077 (June 19, 1989) (exempt organization's participation in a joint venture with a for-profit partner will not affect its exempt status given that exempt organization will hold "a majority interest" and the partnership agreement gives the exempt organization "exclusive discretion in the management and control" of the joint venture); PLR 8936077 (June 19, 1989) (exempt organization's participation in a joint venture with a for-profit partner will not affect its exempt status given that it will maintain "control over" the joint venture by holding "a great majority" of the joint venture equity).

48. See, for example, Rev. Rul. 98-15 (March 4, 1998); PLR 9637050 (June 18, 1996).

49. See PLR 9616005 (Dec. 19, 1995); PLR 9518014 (Feb. 1, 1995); PLR 9352030 (Oct. 8, 1993); PLR 9323030 (March 16, 1993); PLR 9319044 (Feb. 18, 1993); PLR 9318033 (Feb. 8, 1993); PLR 9308034 (Nov. 30, 1992); PLR 9105031 (Nov. 6, 1990); PLR 9105029 (Nov. 6, 1990); PLR 8945063 (Aug. 17, 1989); PLR 8943050 (July 31, 1989); PLR 8925052 (March 28, 1989); PLR 8727080 (April 10, 1987); PLR 8717057 (Jan. 28, 1987); PLR 8531069 (May 10, 1985); PLR 8206093 (Nov. 10, 1981). Indeed, the Service has previously issued guidance indicating that sufficient control could exist when the exempt participant maintained less than a 50% stake in managing the joint venture. See, for example, PLR 9122061 (March 6, 1991) (approving a joint venture in which the exempt organization held 44% of the director slots but board decisions uniformly required 66% approval for adoption and the exempt organization was responsible for day-to-day management of the facility); PLR 8909036 (Dec. 7, 1988) (approving a joint venture in which the exempt participant had only a 40% interest on the management committee and veto power over the assumption of debt by the joint venture).

50. See *St. David's Health Care System*, 2003 U.S. App. Lexis at *26–*27 ("[As] the Government argues, there are reasons to doubt that the partnership documents provide *St. David's* with sufficient control" because, among other things, "St. David's does not control a majority of the Board.")

51. *Redlands Surgical Services*, 113 T.C. at 80–81 (concluding that, in the absence of an outright voting majority on the part of the exempt organization, the court will "look to the binding commitments" between the nonprofit and for-profit participants "to ascertain whether other specific powers or rights conferred upon" the nonprofit entity "might compensate or mitigate for its lack of majority control.").

52. The Service has explicitly stated that it will apply the same control analysis in analyzing joint ventures to form PHOs, MSOs, and other integrated delivery systems as it does in analyzing clinical joint ventures. FY95 CPE Text at 155, 158. Although the Service initially seemed to suggest that physician representation on the board of a PHO or MSO should not exceed 20%, Service representatives have publicly abandoned this approach and conceded that the analysis to be applied in analyzing control of a PHO or MSO is identical to that applied in evaluating clinical joint ventures. Michael W. Peregrine and Bernadette M. Broccolo, *PHO Tax Update*, 11 EOTR 1015, 1020 (May 1995); FY95 CPE Text at 155,158.

53. *Redlands Surgical Services*, 113 T.C. at 80–81.

54. *Redlands Surgical Services*, 113 T.C. at 79–84.

55. *Redlands Surgical Services*, 113 T.C. at 84.

56. *Redlands Surgical Services*, 113 T.C. at 84.

57. *Redlands Surgical Services*, 113 T.C. at 87.

58. *St. David's Health Care System*, 2002 U.S. Dist. Lexis at * 21.

59. *St. David's Health Care System*, 2002 U.S. Dist. Lexis at * 20.

60. PLR 9645018 (Aug. 9, 1996); PLR 9637050 (June 18, 1996); PLR 9231047 (May 5, 1992); PLR 9233037 (May 20, 1992); PLR 9021050 (Feb. 26, 1990).

61. GCM 39862 (Nov. 21, 1991).

62. Thomas K. Hyatt and Bruce R. Hopkins, *The Law of Tax-Exempt Healthcare Organizations* (2nd ed. 2001) ("Hyatt & Hopkins") at 60. See also PLR 39862 (Nov. 21, 1981) ("The proscription against inurement generally applies to a distinct class of private interests —

typically persons who, because of their particular relationship with an organization, have opportunity to control or influence its activities.").

63. Rev. Rul. 97-21 (April 21, 1997).

64. See, for example, Rev. Rule 98-15 (March 4, 1998); GCM 39732 (Nov. 4, 1987); PLR 9035072 (June 7, 1990); PLR 9308034 (Nov. 30, 1992); PLR 9323030 (March 16, 1993); PLR 9318033 (Feb. 8, 1993); PLR 9345057 (Aug. 20, 1993); PLR 9645018 (Aug. 9, 1996); PLR 9637050 (June 18, 1996); PLR 9709014 (Nov. 26, 1996); PLR 9319044 (Feb. 18, 1993) ; PLR 8638131 (June 30, 1986); PLR 8206093 (Nov. 10, 1981); PLR 8715039 (Jan. 13, 1987); PLR 8531069 (May 10, 1985); FY95 CPE Text at 156-157; Hospital Audit Guidelines § 334.4.

65. GCM 39732 (Nov. 4, 1987); PLR 9035072 (June 7, 1990); PLR 9345057 (Aug. 20, 1993); PLR 9352030 (Oct. 8, 1993); PLR 9352030 (Oct. 8, 1993); PLR 9319044 (Feb. 18, 1993) ; PLR 9518014 (Feb. 1, 1995);); PLR 9637050 (June 18, 1996); PLR 9645018 (Aug. 9, 1996); PLR 8945063 (Aug. 17, 1989); PLR 8909036 (Dec. 7, 1988); PLR 9021050 (Feb. 26, 1990); PLR 8727080 (April 10, 1987); PLR 8531069 (May 10, 1985); PLR 8506102 (Nov. 16, 1984); FY95 CPE Text at 156-157; Service Announcement 92-83 (May 31, 1992) ("Hospital Audit Guidelines") § 334.4.

66. *Redlands Surgical Services*, 113 T.C. at 83; PLR 9035072 (June 7, 1990); PLR 9323030 (March 16, 1993); PLR 9318033 (Feb. 8, 1993); PLR 8833038 (May 20, 1988); FY95 CPE Text at 156–157.

67. PLR 9323030 (March 16, 1993); PLR 9345057 (Aug. 20, 1993); PLR 9319044 (Feb. 18, 1993); PLR 9318033 (Feb. 8, 1993); PLR 8206093 (Nov. 10, 1981); PLR 8936077 (June 19, 1989). Hospital Audit Guidelines § 334.4.

68. PLR 9035072 (June 7, 1990); PLR 9035072 (June 7, 1990); PLR 9323030 (March 16, 1993); PLR 9345057 (Aug. 20, 1993); PLR 9637050 (June 18, 1996). Hospital Audit Guidelines § 334.4.

69. PLR 9319044 (Feb. 18, 1993) (exempt hospital has right to buy out partner's interest in joint venture after five years); PLR 8806057 (Nov. 17, 1987) (exempt hospital's participation in a joint venture with a for-profit partner will not affect its exempt status, given that the Hospital "shall have the option to purchase any or all equipment, supplies, and other assets of the partnership"); Williamsburg Ruling.

70. PLR 9709014 (Nov. 26, 1996); PLR 9352030 (Oct. 8, 1993).

71. PLR 9709014 (Nov. 26, 1996).

72. Hospital Audit Guidelines § 333.4; FY95 CPE Text at 156–157; GCM 39732 (Nov. 4, 1987).

73. Hospital Audit Guidelines § 333.4; FY95 CPE Text at 156–157.

74. Hospital Audit Guidelines § 333.4; FY95 CPE Text at 156–157.

75. Hospital Audit Guidelines § 333.4; FY95 CPE Text at 156–157.

76. GCM 39862 (Nov. 21, 1991) ("One of the more troubling characteristics of the arrangements at issue is the complete lack of symmetry in upside opportunities and downside risks for the physician investors," that is, "most of the downside risk" is borne by the exempt hospital while the physician investors receive "tremendous reward potential" with "very little downside risk."); FY95 CPE Text at 156–157.

77. PLR 9709014 (Nov. 26, 1996); PLR 9352030 (Oct. 8, 1993).

78. Rev. Rul. 98-15 (March 4, 1998); *Redlands Surgical Services*, 113 T.C. at 83.

79. *Redlands Surgical Services*, 113 T.C. at 89; PLR 9645018 (Aug. 9, 1996); PLR 8817039 (Jan. 29, 1988). Nonetheless, commercially reasonable mutually binding covenants not to compete with the joint venture are not prohibited. PLR 9318033 (Feb. 8, 1993).

80. GCM 39862 (Nov. 21, 1991) ("[T]he private benefits conferred on the physician-investors by the instant revenue stream joint ventures are direct and substantial, not incidental. If for any reason these benefits should be found not to constitute inurement, they nonetheless exceed the bounds of prohibited private benefit). See also PLR 9231047 (May 5, 1992); PLR 9233037 (May 20, 1992).

81. Gerald M. Griffith, *Refining Joint Venture Control Requirements: St. David's v. Goliath*, EOTR (August 2002) at 255, 257.

82. IRC §§ 511(a), 512(a)(1); Treas. Reg. §§ 1.511-1, 1.511-2(a)(1)(i). As noted above, for purposes of this chapter, we assume that the hospital's exemption is predicated upon § 501(c)(3).

83. IRC § 512(c); Treas. Reg. § 1.512(c)-1. See also *Service Bolt & Nut Co. v. Commissioner*, 724 F.2d 519, 522-523 (6th Cir. 1983); Rev. Rul. 79-222 (Jan. 1, 1979); PLR 9703026 (Oct. 29, 1996). Income to a 501(c)(3) organization from an S corporation is automatically deemed to be unrelated business income. IRC § 512(e).

84. Treas. Reg. § 1.513-1(d)(1).

85. Treas. Reg. § 1.513-1(d)(2); *United States v. American College of Physicians*, 475 U.S. 834, 847-848 (1986).

86. Treas. Reg. § 1.513-1(d)(3).

87. Treas. Reg. § 1.513-1(d)(3).

88. IRC § 513(a); Treas. Reg. § 1.513-1(e)(2). There has been some debate as to whether staff physicians in private practice are "members" of a hospital. Compare *St. Luke's Hospital of Kansas City*, 494 F. Supp. 85, 92-93 (W.D. Mo. 1980) (physicians on a hospital's medical staff are "members" within the meaning of IRC § 513(a)(2)) with Rev. Rul. 85-109 (stating that the Service disagrees with and will not abide by the court's conclusion in *St. Luke's Hospital of Kansas City v. U.S.* that staff physicians in private practice are "members" of the hospital for purposes of IRC § 513).

89. Rev. Rul. 68-376; PLR 8246018 (Aug. 20, 1982); PLR 8206093 (Nov. 10, 1981). See also *Carle Foundation v. United States*, 611 F.2d 1192, 1199 (7th Cir. 1979) (describing the foregoing rulings).

90. Rev. Rul. 69-268; Rev. Rul. 69-269.

91. Hyatt & Hopkins at § 24.5.

92. PLR 8531069 (May 10, 1985); PLR 8638131 (June 30, 1986); PLR 8709051 (Dec. 3, 1986)l; PLR 8715039 (Jan. 13,1987); PLR 8807012 (Oct. 28, 1987); PLR 8806057 (Nov. 17, 1987); PLR 8817039 (Jan. 29, 1988); PLR 8936077 (June 19, 1989); 8941006 (June 29, 1989); PLR 8946067 (Aug. 24, 1989); PLR 9204048 (Oct. 30, 1991); PLR 9407022 (Nov. 22, 1993); PLR 9709014 (Nov. 26, 1996).

93. PLR 9122061 (March 6, 1991); PLR 9105029 (Nov. 6, 1990); PLR 8833038 (May 20, 1988)

94. PLR 8925052 (March 28, 1989).

95. PLR 8717057 (Jan. 28, 1987).

96. PLR 9518014 (Feb. 1, 1995).

97. PLR 8727080 (April 10, 1987).

98. PLR 9318033 (Feb. 8, 1993); PLR 9308034 (Nov. 30, 1992).

99. PLR 9319044 (Feb. 18, 1993).

100. PLR 8903060 (Oct. 25, 1988); PLR 8432014 (April 9, 1984).

101. PLR 9035072 (June 7, 1990).

102. PLR 9323030 (March 16, 1993).

103. PLR 9352030 (Oct. 8, 1993).

104. PLR 8909036 (Dec. 7, 1988).

105. 8945063 (Aug. 17, 1989); PLR 8943050 (July 31,1989); PLR 8934089 (May 31, 1985).

106. PLR 9645018 (Aug. 9, 1996); PLR 9637050 (June 18,1996).

107. PLR 9722042 (March 7, 1997); PLR 9721031 (Feb. 26, 1997); PLR 9714011 (Dec. 24, 1996); PLR 9651047 (Sept. 24, 1996).

108. PLR 9739036 (June 30, 1997). See also PLR 9837031 (June 15, 1988).

109. FY95 CPE Text at 159–160.

110. FY95 CPE Text at 159–160.

111. FY95 CPE Text at 159–160.

112. IRC §§ 512(a)(1), 512(b)(10), 512(b)(12); Treas. Reg. §§ 1.512(a)-1(a)-(c), 1.512(b)-1(g)-(h).

113. IRC § 512(b)(6).

114. IRC § 512(b)(6); Treas. Reg. § 1.512(b)-1(e)(1), 1.512(b)-1(g)-(h).

115. An exempt hospital can create a nonprofit corporate subsidiary to participate in a joint venture activity. Moreover, if the nonprofit subsidiary qualifies for tax-exempt status, it affords the same principal benefit as a Flow-Through Entity: distributions from the joint venture will not be subject to taxation prior to or upon receipt by the exempt hospital. Nonetheless, one substantial impediment typically precludes use of such a nonprofit subsidiary in lieu of a Flow-Through Entity. The nonprofit subsidiary must establish compliance with the community benefit standard (or another basis for exemption) without reference to the charitable and other exempt activities conducted by its exempt parent. *Redlands Surgical Services*, 113 T.C. at 87 (citing *Harding Hospital v. United States*, 505 F.2d 1068 (6th Cir. 1974)). Given the limited scope of and lack of indigent care furnished in connection with many joint venture activities, this requirement may be prohibitive.

116. *Moline Properties v. Commissioner*, 319 U.S. 436, 438 (1943); *Greer v. Commissioner*, 334 F.2d 20, 23 (5th Cir. 1985); PLR 9349032 (Sept. 17, 1993); PLR 9308047 (Dec. 4, 1992); PLR 9105028 (Feb. 1, 1991); GCM 39,326 (Jan. 17, 1985). For discussion of the Service's position as to when a subsidiary is deemed to be established for a legitimate business purpose and treated as a distinct entity, see GCM 35598 (Jan. 23, 1987) and GCM 39326 (Jan. 17, 1985). For a discussion of the use of a subsidiary to convey indirect private inurement, see PLR 9819046 (Feb. 11, 1998), GCM 39646 (June 30, 1987), and GCM 39598 (Jan. 23, 1987).

117. PLR 9349032 (Sept. 17, 1993); PLR 9308047 (Dec. 4, 1992).

118. IRC §§ 511(a), 512(a)(1); Treas. Reg. §§ 1.511-1, 1.511-2(a)(1)(i). As noted above, for purposes of this chapter, we assume that the Hospital's exemption is predicated upon § 501(c)(3).

119. IRC § 512(b)(1); PLR 9349032 (Sept. 17, 1993); PLR 9308047 (Dec. 4, 1992).

120. IRC § 512(b)(13). This will be true even when the joint venture is structured as a Flow-Through Entity.

121. IRC § 512(b)(13).

122. See, for example, FTC Premerger Notification Office, Formal Interpretation 15 (March 2001) ("Formal Interpretation 15") at 4.

123. See, for example, Formal Interpretation 15 at 4. Note that the contribution of intellectual property to a joint venture is deemed the contribution of a business for purposes of triggering the HSR requirement. Formal Interpretation 15 at 4–5.

124. 16 C.F.R. § 801.40(c).

125. Corporate stock is almost invariably deemed to be a security. See *Landreth Timber Co. v. Landreth*, 471 U.S. 681, 692 (1985). So are limited partnership interests. *L&B Hosp. Ventures, Inc. v. Healthcare Int'l*, 894 F.2d 150, 151 (5th Cir. 1990); Carter G. Bishop & Daniel S. Kleinberger, *Limited Liability Companies: Tax and Business Law* (2002) ("Limited Liability Companies") § 11.03[1][c] n.106 (citing cases in which limited partnerships are deemed to be "securities" for purposes of the Securities Act). Although there are credible grounds to contend that LLC membership interests should rarely qualify as a security, the law is sufficiently ambiguous that a joint venture must assume that such interests would be deemed a security. Limited Liability Companies § 11.03[1]. Finally, although general partnership interests are deemed to be exempt from the definition of a security in many contexts, prudence suggests that it must be assumed that such interests might be deemed security interests in a joint venture context. *Williamson v. Tucker*, 645 F.2d 404, 424 (5th Cir. 1981).

CHAPTER 9

Operating the Joint Venture

INTRODUCTION

Federal fraud and abuse laws, tax laws, antitrust laws, securities laws, and Medicare certification requirements place numerous restrictions on the ongoing operations of hospital joint ventures. This chapter addresses the pertinent compliance concerns in each of the foregoing areas and suggests safeguards for joint venture operations so as to promote ongoing compliance with federal law.

FRAUD AND ABUSE ISSUES

Anti-Kickback Law

OIG Concern

When assessing whether a joint venture among health care providers serves as a vehicle to transfer remuneration to induce the referral and promotion of Federal Program business, rather than as a legitimate business venture, the OIG closely scrutinizes the manner in which the joint venture is operated.[1] In most cases, the OIG will focus on whether (1) the joint venture attracts substantial business and referrals from those other than Business Source Investors, (2) the joint venture's services are available to those other than Business Source Investors, and (3) the joint venture ensures that all ancillary agreements with Business Source Investors are commercially reasonable and do not include a premium for the investor to generate Federal Program business for the joint venture or fellow investors.

For joint ventures involving operation of an ASC, the OIG's concerns vary slightly. In such circumstances, the OIG is more concerned that (1) joint venture activities are limited to furnishing ASC-Approved Procedures, (2) patients are made aware of a referring physician's ownership interest, (3) the joint venture ensures that all ancillary agreements with Business Source Investors are commercially reasonable and do not include a premium for the investor to generate Federal Program business for the joint venture or fellow investors, and (4) the investing hospital (if any) does not require or encourage employed or staff physicians to refer patients to, furnish items or services to, or generate business for the ASC.

Regardless of the type of joint venture, safeguards governing joint venture operations can be adopted to (1) protect the joint venture arrangement under an Anti-Kickback Law safe harbor provision or (2) otherwise minimize the risk that the OIG would perceive the joint venture as a means to channel impermissible remuneration to sources of Federal Program business.

Safe Harbor Protection

Investment Interests Safe Harbor The Investment Interests Safe Harbor protection imposes at least four restrictions on joint venture operations. Each restriction is addressed in turn.

First, the OIG requires that no more than 40% of the joint venture's gross revenue related to the furnishing of health care items and services in the previous fiscal year or previous 12-month period may come from referrals or business otherwise generated from investors.[2] This provision is designed to ensure that safe harbor protection is afforded only (1) to those joint ventures that are capable of securing referrals from independent practitioners and (2) when joint venture profit distributions will be dispersed to "a wider group" than those generating business for the joint venture.[3] The joint venture may use any reasonable accounting method to assess compliance with this standard so long as the method is used consistently.[4] In applying the 40% limitation, investment interests held by an entity will be deemed to be held by the entity and imputed proportionally to its investors and beyond until all interests are allotted to individuals.[5]

Second, neither the joint venture nor any investor may market or furnish the joint venture's items or services (or those of another joint venture as part of a cross referral agreement) to passive investors differently than to noninvestors.[6] In light of this restriction, the OIG contends that the joint venture (1) "may not use a separate marketing approach or provide a different level of service to passive investors as opposed to noninvestors," (2) may not appeal to an investor's status as an investor when marketing the joint venture, and (3) "may not offer special arrangements to investors that are not available or are offered on different terms to non-investors."[7] These restrictions collectively ensure that the joint venture markets and offers its services broadly to the public and does not disparately focus on marketing to investors.

Third, the joint venture is prohibited from encouraging or requiring investors to divest their ownership interest in the joint venture if they cease to practice or fail to maintain an "acceptable" level of Federal Program referrals or otherwise generate a sufficient amount of Federal Program business for the joint venture or fellow investors.[8] According to the OIG, joint venture distributions should be a return for capital placed at risk by an investor, and the appropriate return for such capital does not vary depending upon the investor's professional endeavors.

Joint ventures meeting the foregoing requirements are eligible for protection under Investment Interests Safe Harbor provisions so long as the remaining safe harbor requirements relating to investor selection and distributions are met.[9] The safe harbor, however, will only protect payments from the joint venture to an investor, payments that qualify as a "return on investment" (e.g., a dividend, interest payment, or other distribution).[10] Under no circumstance will the safe harbor protect other types of direct or indirect payments made to investors or others who might refer patients to, furnish items or services for, or generate business for the joint venture or fellow investors. Rather, such other payments must be analyzed independently for protection under a separate safe harbor scutiny.[11] The most pertinent safe harbors will likely be those for payments in connection with leases, employment agreements, and other personal services agreements.[12] The specific requirements for these safe harbors are described in Chapter 2.[13]

ASC Safe Harbor The ASC Safe Harbor imposes at least seven restrictions on joint venture operations. Each such restriction is addressed, in turn, below.

First, the ASC must be certified by Medicare.[14] This requirement is designed to ensure that the joint venture facility is truly an ASC.

Second, all ancillary services for Federal Program beneficiaries performed by the joint venture must be "directly and integrally related" to "primary" procedures performed at the ASC, and must not be separately billed to a Federal Program.[15] Thus, the safe harbor will not protect distributions from "ancillary services joint ventures married to ASCs."[16]

Third, patients referred to the ASC joint venture by investors must be "fully informed of the investor's investment interest."[17] According to the OIG, this provision is designed to protect "patient freedom of choice" and "informed decision making."[18]

Fourth, the ASC joint venture and any hospital or physician investor must treat Federal Program beneficiaries in a nondiscriminatory manner.[19] This provision does not prevent a physician from refusing to take on new patients, so long as such refusal applies to all private-pay, self-pay, and Federal Program beneficiaries.[20] Moreover, an ASC is not required to make an affirmative showing that its payer case mix precisely reflects that prevailing in its service area.[21] Rather, the ASC and investing practitioners are precluded from treating Federal Program beneficiaries in a disparate manner from other patients. This requirement is designed to promote access to care by Federal Program beneficiaries and ensure that the cost-efficiencies associated with the performance of surgical services in the ASC setting are passed on to Federal Programs.[22]

Fifth, the ASC must have exclusive use of its operating room and recovery room space, and the investing hospital must not include any costs associated with the joint venture ASC (including operating or development costs) on its cost report or any claim for payment from a Federal Program (unless such costs are required to be included by a Federal Program).[23]

Sixth, the ASC joint venture must not use space owned by or located in an investing hospital, equipment owned by an investing hospital, or services provided by an investing hospital, unless such transactions comply with all requirements for the Lease Safe Harbor or Personal Services Safe Harbor.[24] Compliance with this safeguard will better ensure that the hospital investor is neither receiving inflated payments from the joint venture in return for promoting patient referrals or business for the joint venture or joint venture investors, nor providing the joint venture with items or services at below-market rates in return for Federal Program business from physician investors.

Finally, as noted above, the hospital must not be in a position to make referrals to the joint venture.[25] As further noted above, a hospital will generally be deemed a referral source for an ASC joint venture so as to preclude safe harbor protection.[26] Nonetheless, OIG Advisory Opinions suggest that arrangements that otherwise meet the ASC Safe Harbor requirements will pose minimal risk of fraud and abuse if appropriate measures are taken to constrain the hospital's ability to refer patients to the ASC joint venture. Safeguards would include: (1) the hospital refraining from encouraging employed, contractor, or staff physicians to refer patients to the joint venture ASC or joint venture investors, (2) refraining from tracking referrals from these physicians to the joint venture ASC or joint venture investors, (3) refraining from directly or indirectly predicating compensation to these physicians on referrals to the joint venture ASC or ASC investors, and (4) informing these physicians of the foregoing policies at least annually.[27]

Joint ventures meeting the foregoing requirements are eligible for protection under the ASC Safe Harbor so long as the remaining safe harbor requirements relating to investor selection and distributions are met.[28] Nonetheless, the ASC Safe Harbor, like the Investment Interests Safe Harbor, will only protect payments from the joint venture to an investor, payments that qualify as a "return on investment" (e.g., a dividend, interest payment, or other distribution). Under no circumstance will the safe harbor protect other types of direct or indirect payments to investors (or entity's controlled by investors) or others who might refer patients to, furnish items or services for, or generate business for the joint venture or fellow investors. Rather, such other payments must be analyzed independently for protection under a separate safe harbor.[29] The most pertinent safe harbors will likely be the safe harbor for payments in connection with leases or personal services agreements. The specific requirements for these safe harbors are described in Chapter 2.[30]

Safeguards to Lower Risk for Joint Ventures Outside a Safe Harbor

Investment Interests Generally Even when a joint venture will not be operated in accord with all requirements to qualify for safe harbor protection, certain safeguards governing business operations can be adopted to reduce the regulatory risk associated with the joint venture.

First, joint venture representatives should document that a substantial portion of the joint venture's revenues relating to the furnishing of health care items and services are generated by individuals who are not investors. As noted above, the OIG believes that a joint venture capable of competing for referrals and business on the open market in terms of quality and price is less likely to be a sham conduit through which to channel payment for Federal Program business.[31] Thus, a joint venture can reduce the risk of an enforcement action by ensuring that a substantial proportion of its health care revenues are from noninvestors. The degree of protection will be further augmented where the joint venture is able to show that it markets its services similarly to noninvestors and passive investors.

Second, the joint venture should refrain from pressuring investors to generate Federal Program business and refrain from otherwise treating investors in a disparate manner based upon the amount of Federal Program business they generate.[32] To that end, joint venture representatives should refrain from tracking (or having others track) the volume or value of referrals from, items or services furnished by, or business generated by investors and in any way pressuring investors to increase such activity or divest their interests.[33]

Finally, operating arrangements (e.g., space leases, equipment leases, or personal services arrangements) should be carefully crafted. Often it may not be feasible to structure such arrangements in accord with the literal requirements of the Lease Safe Harbor or Personal Services Safe Harbor. Even absent safe harbor compliance, however, the risk of fraud and abuse associated with such arrangements can be substantially reduced in the eyes of the OIG where the parties execute a written agreement in which (1) the space, equipment, and services furnished to the joint venture are clearly defined and (2) the terms of the arrangement are documented to be commercially reasonable (i.e., indicative of similar transactions between parties negotiating at arm's-length).

Investment Interests in an ASC   Even when a joint venture will not be operated in accord with all requirements to qualify for protection under the ASC Safe Harbor, certain safeguards governing ASC business operations can be adopted to reduce the regulatory risk associated with the joint venture.

First, lease arrangements and personal service arrangements between the joint venture and its hospital investors (and nonhospital investors) that do not fully comply with all safe harbor requirements for such agreements can still be structured in a manner that minimizes the risk of Federal Program abuse. Although specific safeguards must be developed on a case-by-case basis, depending upon the nature of the agreement, such safeguards generally ensure that the terms of the arrangement (1) are memorialized, (2) run for a fixed term, and (3) are equivalent to arrangements that would be negotiated by two parties (with no other financial dealings between them) acting at arm's length and are in no way predicated upon the level of Federal Program business or referrals generated by or for either party.

Second, the mere fact that the hospital investor is in a position to generate referrals or business for the joint venture will not lead to a high risk of abuse in the eyes of the OIG so long as the investing hospital agrees in writing that it will (1) not track referrals to the joint venture, the hospital, or other joint venture investors, (2) neither compensate nor encourage staff or employed physicians to refer patients to the joint venture or joint venture investors, and (3) inform staff and employed physicians of these policies in writing no less than annually.[34]

Third, a substantial portion of each physician investor's income should come from the performance of ASC-approved procedures so as to demonstrate that the facility truly is an "extension" of each physician-investor's office. Once the ASC is operational, the physician-investor should perform a substantial proportion of his or her ASC-approved procedures there.

Stark Law

As noted in Chapter 2, the Stark Law precludes a joint venture from billing Medicare for any DHS it furnishes pursuant to a referral by a physician with whom it has an unexcepted direct or indirect financial relationship. As further noted, if a joint venture bills Medicare in violation of this restriction, it risks liability in the form of Medicare overpayments, civil money penalties, and potential false claims. Thus, once joint venture representatives determine that they will be providing services that could qualify as DHS under the Stark Law, the joint venture should adopt safeguards to (1) identify those physicians with whom it maintains a nonexempt financial relationship, (2) inform those physicians that they are generally precluded from referring Medicare patients to the joint venture for DHS, and (3) identify any improper DHS claims generated by the joint venture before the claim is submitted to Medicare.

Determining Whether the Joint Venture Furnishes DHS

A joint venture need only adopt safeguards to ensure that it bills Medicare in compliance with the Stark Law if the joint venture furnishes DHS. As noted above, DHS includes inpatient hospital services, outpatient hospital services, clinical laboratory services, physical therapy, occupational therapy, speech-language pathology services, radiology and certain other imaging services, radiation therapy services and supplies, durable medical equipment and supplies, home health services, outpatient prescription drugs, prosthetics, orthotics, and parenteral and enteral nutrients, equipment, and supplies.[35] If joint venture representatives are uncertain as to whether an item or service constitutes DHS, they can consult the list of DHS billing codes maintained (and updated annually) by CMS.[36]

Identifying Physicians with Whom the Joint Venture has a Direct or Indirect Financial Relationship

Assuming the joint venture will furnish DHS to Medicare beneficiaries (and bill for such DHS), joint venture representatives should exercise due diligence to identify the names of those physicians maintaining a "financial relationship" with the joint venture. Such financial relationships will typically arise through one of the following scenarios.

Investor Physicians A physician taking equity or secured debt in a joint venture will incur a nonexempt "financial relationship" with the joint venture under the Stark Law unless either of the following is met:

- The joint venture is a hospital at which the investing physician maintains staff privileges, and the investing physician's investment interest is in the entire hospital (not a mere subdivision or department of the facility). (Please note that § 507 of P.L. 108-173 makes this exception unavailable until May 18, 2005 for "specialty hospitals" outside of Puerto Rico unless they were in operation nor under development as of November 18, 2003 and have not done any of the following since that date: (1) increased the number of physician investors, (2) added certain categories of new clinical services, (3) added bed capacity in contravention of certain restrictions, or (4) violates other requirements to be designated by the Secretary.

For purposes of this restriction, a "specialty hospital" is one "primarily or exclusively" engaged in treating patients with a cardiac or orthopedic condition, undergoing surgery, or receiving any other "specialized category of services that the Secretary designates as "inconsistent with the purpose of permitting physician ownership and investment interests in a hospital" under the "Whole Hospital Investment Interest Exception.");[37] or

- The joint venture furnishes DHS to the referring physician's patient in a rural area and "substantially all" of the joint venture's DHS is furnished to residents of a rural area.[38]

Absent either of the foregoing exceptions, the financial relationship arises regardless of whether the physician holds the equity or secured debt directly (i.e., personally holds an ownership interest in the joint venture) or indirectly (i.e., there is a chain of one or more juridical entities or intermediaries between the physician and the joint venture, and each successive entity between the joint venture to the investor holds an ownership interest in the entity below it).[39] Thus, the investor physician must not refer Medicare patients to the joint venture for DHS, and the joint venture must not bill for any DHS furnished pursuant to a prohibited referral.

Even if one of the foregoing exceptions applies, the analysis is not complete. Specifically, if the investor maintains a financial relationship with the joint venture in the form of a compensation arrangement, that arrangement must be separately analyzed in order to determine whether it generates a financial relationship implicating the Stark Law.

Directly Compensated Physicians Physicians receiving any payment or benefit (in cash or in kind) from the joint venture will be deemed to have a "financial relationship" with the joint venture"[40] unless the arrangement between the joint venture and the Compensated Physician is limited to one or more of the following:

- **A Qualified Personal Services Arrangement:** A qualified personal services arrangement is one which meets each of the following requirements: (1) it is memorialized in an agreement signed by the parties, which runs for a term of at least one year, (2) it covers all services to be furnished between the parties, (3) the aggregate services do not exceed those "reasonable and necessary" for the principal's "legitimate business purposes," (4) the agreement would be commercially reasonable in an arm's-length transaction between parties who make no referrals, and (5) the compensation paid in connection with the agreement is "set in advance" (whether in aggregate or on a per-use basis) at fair market value and does not vary during the agreement based on the volume or value of business between the parties.[41]

- **A Qualified Employment Arrangement:** A qualified employment arrangement is one that meets each of the following requirements: (1) it covers identifiable services to be performed by the physician, (2) the agreement would be commercially reasonable in an arm's-length transaction between parties who make no referrals, and (3) the compensation paid in connection with the agreement is "set in advance" (whether in aggregate or on a per-use basis) at fair market value and does not vary during the agreement based on the volume or value of business between the parties.[42]

- **A Qualified Physician Purchase Arrangement:** A qualified physician purchase arrangement is one in which a physician pays fair market value for items or services actually furnished.[43]

- **A Qualified Fair-Market-Value Transaction:** A qualified fair-market-value transaction is one which meets each of the following requirements: (1) it provides for the sale of items or services from a physician or his or her qualified group practice, (2) it is memorialized in an agreement signed by the parties, which runs for a fixed term and specifies all services furnished and compensation paid in connection with the arrangement, (3) it is "commercially reasonable" in scope and duration so as to further the "legitimate business purposes" of the parties, (4) it does not violate the Anti-Kickback Law or involve the counseling or promotion of a business arrangement or activity which violates Federal law, (5) the compensation paid in connection with the agreement is "set in advance" (whether in aggregate or on a per-use basis) at fair market value and does not vary during the agreement based on the volume or value of business between the parties.[44]

- **Waiver of Fees for Erroneous Services:** Forgiveness of amounts owed for inaccurate or mistakenly performed tests or procedures.[45]

- **Correction of Billing Errors:** Correction of minor billing errors.[46]

- **Devices for Specimen Collection:** Non-surgical devices or supplies used to collect transport, process, or store specimens.[47]

- **Qualified Items Relating to Communication of Test Orders or Test Results:** Certain devices, or supplies used solely to order tests or communicate test results.[48]

- **Qualified Health Plan Payments:** Certain payments by health plans for physician services furnished to plan beneficiaries.[49]

In some cases, the physician might also be a joint venture investor. Thus, even if one of the foregoing exceptions is applicable, separate inquiry must be made as to whether the physician's investment interest may independently preclude DHS referrals.

Indirectly Compensated Physicians CMS will deem a physician to have a "financial relationship" with the joint venture in the form of an "indirect compensation arrangement" if (1) there is an unbroken chain of one or more persons between the physician and the joint venture, (2) the compensation received by the physician from the person with whom he or she has a direct relationship varies with the volume or value of referrals or other business the physician generates for the joint venture, and (3) the joint venture has actual knowledge or acts in reckless disregard or deliberate ignorance of the fact that the physician's compensation varies in such a manner.[50] Consequently, the physician will be precluded from referring Medicare beneficiaries to the joint venture for DHS, and the joint venture will be precluded from billing for such DHS, unless one of the following exceptions applies:

- **Qualified Indirect Compensation Arrangement:** The arrangement between the joint venture and Compensated Physician is structured so that (1) compensation received by the referring physician is commercially reasonable fair market value for identifiable services and items actually provided not taking into account the volume or value of referrals or other business generated by the referring physician for the joint venture, (2) unless it is an employment arrangement, it is memorialized in a writing signed by the parties, which specifies the items or services covered, and (3) it does not violate the Anti-Kickback Law or any laws or regulations governing billing or claims submission.[51]

- **Personally Furnished DHS:** The Compensated Physician "personally furnishes" any DHS provided at the joint venture to the patients he or she refers.[52]

- **Qualified DHS:** The DHS furnished to the Medicare beneficiary is limited to the following types of DHS:

  - Clinical laboratory services furnished in an ASC, ESRD facility, or hospice and included in the ASC rate, ESRD composite rate, or the per-diem hospice charge.[53]

  - Designated dialysis-related outpatient prescription drugs administered or dispensed by an ESRD facility.[54]

  - Designated preventive screening tests, immunizations, and vaccines.[55]

  - Eyeglasses and contact lenses covered by Medicare when furnished to patients following cataract surgery.[56]

  - Implants (including, without limitation, cochlear implants, intraocular lenses, implanted prosthetic devices, and implanted DME) furnished by the referring physician or a member of his or her group practice and implanted in a surgical procedure performed at the certified ASC where the implant is furnished.[57]

- **Qualified Prepaid Health Plan Services:** The Medicare beneficiary referred to the joint venture is enrolled in to receive (1) a health plan that contracts with CMS pursuant to § 1876 of the Social Security Act, (2) a health care prepayment plan that contracts with CMS pursuant to § 1833(a)(1)(A) of the Social Security Act, (3) a health plan receiving payment on a prepaid basis pursuant to certain demonstration projects authorized under the Social Security Act, (4) an HMO qualified under the Federal HMO Act, or (5) a Medicare+Choice coordinated care plan.[58]

- Rural Services: The joint venture furnishes DHS to the patient in a rural area and "substantially all" of its DHS is furnished to residents of a rural area.[59]

Absent one of the foregoing exceptions, indirectly compensated physician must not refer Medicare patients to the joint venture for DHS, and the joint venture must not bill for any DHS furnished pursuant to a prohibited referral.

Ensuring That Any Improper DHS Claims Are Identified Before Submission to Medicare.

Finally, the joint venture furnishing DHS could develop screens within its billing software to identify Medicare claims arising from a referral from a physician with a financial relationship with the joint venture. This process will be facilitated by the fact that the Medicare physician identifier number for the referring physician is already included on the principal Medicare billing forms (Form CMS 1450 and Form CMS 1500). Claims should be so identified for further review prior to submission in order to determine (1) whether the claim involves the furnishing of DHS and (2) if so, whether one of the foregoing Stark Law exceptions applies. If an improper claim is discovered after money has been collected from the beneficiary, Medicare, or a Medicare Supplemental plan, such payment must be refunded immediately.

Exclusion

As described in Chapter 2, HHS has discretion to exclude a joint venture from participation in a Federal Program if a person acting as an officer, director, agent, or managing employee of the venture has been (1) convicted of certain enumerated crimes relating to health care billing, patient care, substance abuse, patient care, or obstruction of a state or federal investigation, (2) held liable for civil monetary penalties under the Social Security Act, or (3) excluded from participation in a Federal health care program.[60] As further described above, if a joint venture "arranges or contracts" with an individual or entity for the provision of items or services that may be paid for by a Federal Program, and such person "knows or should know" that the individual or entity has been excluded from participation in Federal Programs, HHS may (1) impose a $10,000 civil monetary penalty and assessment of treble damages for each item or service furnished to a federal program beneficiary and (2) exclude such person from participation in Federal Programs.[61]

Consequently, a joint venture directly or indirectly involved in the furnishing of health care services must adopt safeguards to (1) screen potential officers, employees, and contractors for exclusion, (2) periodically screen existing officers, employees, and contractors for exclusion, (3) mandate that officers, employees, and contractors immediately inform the joint venture if they are excluded from Federal Programs, and (4) reserve the right to immediately terminate them upon exclusion.

TAX COMPLIANCE

Compliance with Restrictions on Use of Tax-Exempt Bond Proceeds

Many exempt hospitals rely upon proceeds from "qualified 501(c)(3) bonds" as a source of comparatively low-cost capital for financing capital improvements.[62] The interest paid by the hospital on such bonds is excludable for federal (and often state and local) income tax purposes.[63] Consequently, investors accept a lower interest rate than would be demanded on a taxable investment instrument.[64]

The exclusion of interest payments is predicated upon the exempt hospital's ongoing compliance with several requirements.[65] First, any property financed with bond proceeds must be owned exclusively by the exempt hospital (or a governmental unit).[66] Second, no more than 5% of the "net proceeds" of a bond issue made after 1986 may be devoted to (and payment of the principal or interest on no more than 5% of the net proceeds of an issue may be directly or indirectly related to property put to) a nonqualifying use.[67] A "nonqualifying use" includes (1) any direct or indirect use of bond proceeds by a person other than the hospital and (2) the direct or indirect use of bond proceeds by the exempt hospital for an activity unrelated to its charitable purpose.[68] For purposes of this test, use of property bought or financed with proceeds constitutes the use of proceeds.[69] Third, no more than 2% of the proceeds from the issuance can be used to finance the costs of the issuance itself (e.g., attorney's fees, underwriter's fees, accountant's fees), and use of proceeds in this manner counts against the 5% limitation for noncharitable use: IRC § 147(g)(1); Treas. Reg. § 1.145-2.

When an exempt hospital fails to abide by the foregoing restrictions, the Service can impose sanctions on the bondholders as well as the hospital. The bondholders may be required to pay tax on interest payments on the bonds retroactive to the date of issuance.[70] The hospital will be treated as receiving unrelated business income in an amount equal to the fair market rental value of the bond-financed property.[71] Moreover, the hospital will be precluded from deducting interest on the bond issue against the unrelated business income from the bond-financed property.[72] Ultimately, the hospital's exempt status could be placed at risk.[73] These sanctions can be avoided if certain conditions are met and (1) the bonds are immediately redeemed or (2) the facility is put to a "qualified" charitable use.[74]

Exempt hospitals have little (if any) flexibility to use bond-financed property in connection with joint venture arrangements with for-profit persons. Bond-financed property may not be transferred (via sale, lease, or grant) to such a joint venture absent a redemption of the underlying bond issue.[75] Indeed, even management agreements for bond-financed facilities falling well short of true joint venture arrangements must be structured carefully to avoid any characterization that they give rise to private use of bond proceeds.[76] The Service may be more flexible, however, in permitting a joint venture to use bond-financed facilities if the venture is exclusively between 501(c)(3) exempt entities.

Avoiding Intermediate Sanctions

Although hospital management and the nonhospital joint venture participants bear the direct liability for any intermediate sanctions arising from joint venture transactions, the exempt hospital is best positioned to prevent such transactions from arising in the first instance. Moreover, such action is prudent on the part of the hospital in that excess benefit transactions could still give rise to impermissible private benefit or private inurement that would threaten the hospital's exempt status. Specifically, the hospital must adopt safeguards that address the risk of excess benefit transactions between the hospital and joint venture entity, the joint venture entity and third parties, and the hospital and joint venture participants. The risk of an excess benefit under each scenario will vary depending principally upon whether the exempt hospital participates in the joint venture as an active investor (i.e., a general partner or active LLC member) or a passive investor (i.e., a limited partner, non-managing LLC member, or C corporation shareholder). We address the regulatory risks and appropriate safeguards under each alternative scenario.

Joint Ventures in which the Exempt Hospital Is a General Partner or Active LLC Member

The risk of an excess benefit transaction arising from a joint venture arrangement is greatest when the exempt hospital participates as a general partner or active LLC member. First, the hospital's transactions with the joint venture itself can result in liability if more than 35% of the profit interest in the joint venture is held by disqualified persons or their family members.[77] Second, liability could also result by virtue of contracts between the joint venture and third parties (irrespective of whether the hospital is aware of the contract). As noted above, both the Service and federal courts have taken the position that when an exempt hospital participates in a joint venture as a general partner or managing LLC member, the activities of the joint venture are imputed to the hospital.[78] Thus, when a joint venture contracts with a third party, the contract could be imputed to the general partner. If that third party is a disqualified person with respect to the hospital, an excess benefit transaction could arise (even if the hospital was unaware of the existence or terms of the contract). Third, liability could arise by virtue of an exempt hospital's contract with individuals outside the joint venture arrangement altogether. If the Service does attribute the activities of the joint venture to the exempt hospital, the following persons would become "disqualified persons" with respect to the hospital without ever interacting directly with the hospital:

- Persons whose compensation is "primarily based" on revenues from the joint venture (or a particular "department or function" of the joint venture) that such person controls.

- Persons who share authority to control or determine a "substantial portion" of the joint venture's capital expenditures, operating budget or employee compensation (where they are, in turn, a "substantial portion" of the hospital's expenditures, budget, or compensation).

- Persons who "manage" joint venture activities that represent a substantial portion of the hospital's overall activities, assets, or income.

In order to minimize the threat of an excess benefit transaction under any of the foregoing scenarios, an exempt hospital should adopt a three-part strategy. First, it should ensure that it accurately values and receives appropriate consideration for property, services, or capital furnished to the joint venture itself (both during and after initial capitalization). The hospital must be particularly vigilant when disqualified persons with respect to the hospital collectively maintain 35% control in the joint venture. Therefore, the hospital should consider mandating advance approval prior to the transfer of goods, services, or capital between the hospital and the joint venture. To the extent possible, the hospital should follow those procedures necessary to establish the presumption of reasonableness regarding the transaction.

Second, the exempt hospital should secure authority in the documents governing the joint venture to ensure that the hospital will receive (1) timely advance notice of contracts or transactions that the joint venture proposes to execute and that exceed a fixed dollar amount, (2) that information necessary for the hospital to assess whether the contract poses a credible risk of an excess benefit transaction, and (3) the right to veto such an arrangement prior to execution when, in its discretion, an excess benefit transaction might result.

Third, the exempt hospital should secure authority in the documents governing the joint venture to ensure that joint venture management provide periodic updates identifying those individuals who could be considered to have "substantial influence" in connection with the joint venture. The hospital should also reserve the right to make its own independent review of joint venture records to make its own determinations on this point. If properly utilized, these disclosure and audit rights could prove invaluable to the hospital in identifying individuals who become disqualified persons with respect to the hospital solely by dint of their interaction with the joint venture. Absent such disclosure, the hospital would be hard pressed to identify those individuals who might fall within this subset of its disqualified persons.

Joint Ventures in Which the Exempt Hospital Is a Limited Partner, Passive LLC Member, or C Corporation Shareholder

The risk of an excess benefit transaction arising from a joint venture arrangement is more limited when the exempt hospital participates as a limited partner, nonmanaging LLC member, or corporation shareholder. The hospital's transactions with the joint venture itself can result in liability if more than 35% of the profit interest in the joint venture is held by disqualified persons or their family members.[79] Liability from joint venture contracts and independent hospital contracts with joint venture participants will otherwise arise only if the hospital maintains 50% control of the joint venture. If the hospital maintains such control, it is equated with the joint venture and is effectively treated as if it were an active participant. Thus, contracts between the joint venture and someone who is a disqualified person with respect to the exempt hospital could give rise to intermediate sanctions (even where the hospital is unaware of the contract or its terms). Moreover, joint venture officers, directors, employees, and managers risk becoming disqualified persons with respect to the hospital through their duties with the joint venture.

If the exempt hospital maintains less than 50% control, however, the joint venture's contracts with third parties are less likely to give rise to an excess benefit transaction, unless the hospital affirmatively uses the joint venture as an intermediary (i.e., a conduit) to funnel excess compensation to an otherwise disqualified person. Furthermore joint venture officers, directors, employees, and managers should not automatically be deemed disqualified persons with respect to the hospital solely due to their duties in connection with the joint venture.

If the exempt hospital maintains less than 50% control as a limited partner, nonmanaging LLC member, or shareholder, the joint venture's provision of below-market goods or services to others should not be imputed to the hospital. Similarly, those persons with substantial influence over the joint venture should not automatically become disqualified persons with respect to the hospital. Therefore, the exempt hospital need only be concerned with its direct interactions with the joint venture and ensure that it accurately values and receives appropriate consideration for property, services, or capital furnished to the joint venture itself. (The hospital must be particularly vigilant when disqualified persons with respect to the hospital collectively maintain 35% control in the joint venture.) Therefore, the exempt hospital should consider mandating advance approval prior to the transfer of goods, services, or capital between the hospital and the joint venture. To the extent possible, the hospital should follow those procedures necessary to establish the presumption of reasonableness regarding the transaction. If the hospital maintains 50% control of the joint venture, however, it should adopt the same safeguards as appropriate for general partners and active LLC members.

ANTITRUST COMPLIANCE

Clinical Joint Ventures

A joint venture must maintain general operational safeguards governing interactions with its potential and actual competitors as well as additional safeguards governing interactions with those potential or actual competitors who are joint venture participants. We address each in turn. As a prefatory matter, we also note that a joint venture involved in cooperative research may wish to register under the NRCP in order to secure limitations on liability provided under the Act.

General Safeguards Governing Interaction with Potential and Actual Joint Venture Competitors

The joint venture must establish operational safeguards to ensure that joint venture personnel do not improperly disclose information to actual or potential competitors and this disclosure could serve as the foundation for anticompetitive collusion.[80] Such disclosures must be prevented with respect to third-party competitors as well as joint venture participants who are actual or potential competitors with the joint venture (though disclosure can be made to such investors as reasonably necessary for efficient operation of a procompetitive joint venture).

Safeguards must be particularly strict with respect to information regarding current or future pricing, current or future personnel compensation, or other competitive information which could serve as the basis for anticompetitive collusion.[81] Some allotment may be made, however, for disclosures in connection with (1) a third-party survey of prices and compensation within a given industry or (2) a collective submission of fee information to (and at the request of) purchasers of health care services.[82] Nonetheless, disclosures under either circumstance, should be limited to arrangements that substantially comply with the applicable antitrust safety zone described in Chapter 4.

General Safeguards Governing Interaction with Joint Venture Participants Who Are Potential or Actual Joint Venture Competitors

As noted above, if the joint venture will compete in a highly concentrated market with substantial barriers to timely market entry, joint venture participation by actual or potential competitors will invite heightened scrutiny from DOJ/FTC and should not be considered absent an overriding business interest. If such an arrangement is nonetheless pursued, regulatory risk can be reduced if (1) the joint venture is nonexclusive (i.e., joint venture participants are permitted to—and ideally do—compete with the joint venture), (2) the joint venture is finite in duration, (3) the assets contributed by joint venture participants will not effectively impede their ability to remain in competition with the joint venture, (4) the competing participant's interest in the joint venture is relatively small, and (5) joint venture participants are not required to contribute assets which might otherwise preclude them from competing investor's participation.[83] Regulatory risk can be further reduced to the extent that joint venture participants are restricted in their ability to exercise significant control over daily joint venture operations or competitively significant decisions (such as the collaboration's price and output) and to the extent that joint venture staff are independent of and not directly accountable to the competing participants.[84]

Contract Joint Ventures

The requisite operational safeguards to ensure a Contract Joint Venture's ongoing compliance with federal antitrust laws will vary depending upon whether the joint venture will or will not involve price-fixing arrangements among competing providers. We address both alternatives separately.

Contracting Joint Ventures Involving Price Fixing

Government scrutiny will be greatest in connection with the establishment of Contracting Joint Ventures that prospectively fix prices to be charged by providers for the services provided through the arrangement.[85] There are two general types of safeguards that such joint ventures should adopt and implement in their daily operations.

First, Joint Venture representatives must ensure that there is adequate financial or clinical integration among joint venture participants to achieve efficiencies benefiting consumers, (e.g., quality assurance, reduced administrative costs, economies of scale), and that agreements among participants relating to price or other matters is "reasonably necessary" to realize those efficiencies.[86] Failure to do so will likely render the joint venture illegal *per se*.

The requisite financial integration can be achieved through one of the following arrangements:

- Agreement by the Contracting Joint Venture to provide services to a payor at a "capitated rate."[87]

- Agreement by the Contracting Joint Venture to provide designated services or classes of health services to a health plan for a predetermined percent of premium or revenue from the plan.[88]

- Agreement by the Contracting Joint Venture to provide "significant financial incentives" to its participating providers "as a group" to achieve specified cost-containment goals (e.g., substantial withholds from payments to all participating providers with later distribution predicated upon network-wide realization of specified cost-containment goals or substantial rewards or penalties associated with venture-wide achievement of specified cost or utilization targets).[89]

- Agreement by the Contracting Joint Venture to provide a "complex or extended course of treatment" that requires "substantial coordination of care by different types of providers offering complementary services for a fixed, predetermined amount" and for which the cost can vary greatly.[90]

The requisite form of clinical integration necessary to support a Contracting Joint Venture engaged in price fixing is less clear. Recently, however, the FTC did provide some of the more significant guidance regarding types of clinical integration that might support a price-fixing arrangement. Specifically, the FTC issued an advisory opinion to MedSouth, Inc., concluding that a nonexclusive IPA arrangement in which the IPA negotiated fee-for-service rates with third-party payors would not presently warrant a regulatory enforcement action in light of the significant clinical integration fostered by the IPA.[91] Specifically, the IPA proposed to develop and implement the following mechanisms for clinical integration: (1) establishment of a web-based clinical data record utilized by all IPA members to share medical records, access test results, and transfer physician orders; (2) development and adoption of common clinical protocols for specific diagnoses; (3) development and monitoring of physician performance against clinical benchmarks, and (4) termination of physicians who fail to meet specified quality standards. The FTC concluded that the IPA's ability to negotiate common fee-for-service rates through the nonexclusive IPA was reasonably related to the achievement the procompetitive efficiencies associated with integration. In doing so, the FTC emphasized that the IPA would be nonexclusive and further noted that the IPA would retain an independent consultant who would submit bids on its behalf while preventing the disclosure of competitive information among its members.

Second, the joint venture must adopt safeguards to ensure that it will not obtain sufficient market concentration in any of its component clinical service lines (i.e., hospital care within an integrated network) to permit it to raise prices for the component service.[92] Perhaps the most effective way to do this is to make joint venture participation "nonexclusive" (i.e., permit network providers to furnish their services outside—as well as through—the network).[93] If a Contracting Joint Venture must be exclusive in certain respects, regulatory risk can be reduced to the extent (1) the joint venture maintains a moderate or low market share with respect to the providers in each clinical service subject to the exclusivity requirement, (2) the duration of the exclusivity period is limited, (3) participants are permitted to withdraw from the joint venture with minimal financial penalties or disincentives, and (4) the joint venture does not maintain exclusive arrangements with such a proportion of the practitioners in a given specialty (e.g., obstetricians) or specialized providers (e.g., hospitals) so as to prevent the formation of other Contracting Joint Ventures in the pertinent geographic market.[94]

Contracting Joint Ventures Not Involving Price Fixing

Contracting Joint Ventures which do not involve joint pricing among participating providers pose little risk under federal antitrust laws (e.g., messenger-model PHOs).[95] Typically, participating providers use the Contracting Joint Venture as an independent agent to convey to purchasers the price-related terms the individual provider is willing to accept.[96] DOJ/FTC believe such arrangements raise little concern under federal antitrust law so long as they neither create nor facilitate a collective agreement among participating providers on price or price-related terms.[97] Thus, the joint venture should maintain distinct personnel who are not directly responsible to any member of the Joint Venture. Compensation received by such personnel should not be determined by joint venture members. The joint venture should also maintain separate office space and budget resources that are not dependent upon the approval of any single member. Moreover, the joint venture must adopt safeguards to ensure that joint venture representatives do not (1) disseminate the views or intentions of a participating provider regarding a proposal from/to a purchaser, (2) express opinion on the terms offered by or to be offered to a purchaser, or (3) exercise independent judgment as to whether a given offer is sufficiently attractive to be conveyed to or from a provider.[98]

MEDICARE CERTIFICATION

Joint ventures furnishing clinical services to patients might wish to participate in federal health care programs such as Medicare, Medicaid, Tricare, and the Federal Employees Health Benefits Plan ("FEHBP"). Medicaid participation requirements are codified in state law, and participation in Tricare and FEHBP is negotiated by contract. Participation in the Medicare, however, requires compliance with a number of federal statutory and regulatory requirements. The requirements applicable to the most common types of clinical joint ventures are found in Chapter 6.

ENDNOTES

1. Joint Venture Fraud Alert at 65374.

2. 42 C.F.R. § 1001.952(a)(2)(vi).

3. 56 Fed. Reg. at 35969; OIG Advisory Opinion 98-12 at 4.

4. 56 Fed. Reg. at 35969.

5. 42 C.F.R. § 1001.952(a)(4) (defining the term "investor"); 56 Fed. Reg. at 35967, 35969.

6. 42 C.F.R. § 1001.952(a)(2)(v).

7. 56 Fed. Reg. at 35966.

8. Joint Venture Fraud Alert at 65374.

9. See Chapter 2 for an overview of the other elements of the Investment Interests Safe Harbor.

10. 42 C.F.R. § 1001.952(a); 56 Fed. Reg. 35970-35971.

11. 56 Fed. Reg. 35970-35971.

12. See 42 C.F.R. §§ 1001.952(b) (space rental), 1001.952(c) (equipment rental), 1001.952(d) (personal services agreements), 1001.952(i) (employment agreements).

13. See Chapter 2.

14. 42 C.F.R. § 1001.952(r); 64 Fed. Reg. at 63538.

15. 42 C.F.R. § 1001.952(r)(4)(vi).

16. 64 Fed. Reg. at 63539.

17. 42 C.F.R. § 1001.952(r).

18. 64 Fed. Reg. at 63536.

19. 42 C.F.R. § 1001.952(r)(4)(iv).

20. 64 Fed. Reg. at 63538.

21. 64 Fed. Reg. at 63538.

22. 64 Fed. Reg. at 63538.

23. 42 C.F.R. § 1001.952(r); 64 Fed. Reg. at 63535, 63538.

24. 42 C.F.R. § 1001.952(r)(4)(v); 64 Fed. Reg. at 63538.

25. 42 C.F.R. § 1001.952(r)(4)(viii).

26. 64 Fed. Reg. at 63537.

27. See OIG Advisory Opinion 01-at 10; OIG Advisory Opinion 01-17 at 7; OIG Advisory Opinion 97-5 at 7.

28. See Chapter 2 for an overview of the other elements of the ASC Safe Harbor.

29. 56 Fed. Reg. 35970-35971.

30. See Chapter 2.

31. 56 Fed. Reg. at 35969; OIG Advisory Opinion 98-12 at 4.

32. Joint Venture Fraud Alert at 65374.

33. Joint Venture Fraud Alert at 65374.

34. OIG Advisory Opinion 01-21 at 6; OIG Advisory Opinion 01-17 at 3–4.

35. 42 U.S.C. § 1395nn(h)(6); 42 C.F.R. § 411.351.

36. The list is posted on the CMS website at www.cms.gov. Although the list does not cover billing codes in each category of DHS, it does enumerate the billing codes in those DHS categories most likely to give rise to billing questions.

37. 42 U.S.C. § 1395nn(d)(3); 42 C.F.R. § 411.356(c)(3). If the hospital is located in Puerto Rico, more liberal restrictions apply. Specifically, the Investing Physician need not have privileges there, and his or her investment interest may be in a subdivision or department of the facility. 42 U.S.C. § 1395nn(d)(1); 42 C.F.R. § 411.356(c)(2).

38. 42 U.S.C. § 1395nn(d)(2). For purposes of this exception, the term "rural" means an area designated as rural for purposes of calculating the standardized amount for hospitals located in the area under the Medicare inpatient prospective payment system for acute care hospitals. 42 U.S.C. § 1395nn(d)(2).

39. 42 C.F.R. § 411.354(b).

40. See 42 C.F.R. §§ 411.354(c) (defining "compensation arrangement" to mean the furnishing of "remuneration"), 411.351 (defining "remuneration" to include "any payment or other benefit made directly or indirectly, overtly or covertly, in cash or in kind").

41. 42 C.F.R. § 411.357(d).

42. 42 C.F.R. § 411.357(c).

43. 42 C.F.R. § 411.357(i). See 42 C.F.R. § 411.351 (defining the term "fair market value").

44. 42 C.F.R. §§ 411.357(l), 411.354(d). If the arrangement is for a term of less than one year, it can be renewed any number of times within a year of execution of the first arrangement so long as the terms of the arrangement (including, without limitation, the compensation terms) do not change. 42 C.F.R. § 411.357(l)(2).

45. 42 C.F.R. § 411.351 (defining "remuneration").

46. 42 C.F.R. § 411.351 (defining "remuncration").

47. 42 C.F.R. § 411.351 (defining "remuneration").

48. 42 C.F.R. § 411.351 (defining "remuneration").

49. 42 C.F.R. § 411.351 (defining "remuneration").

50. 42 C.F.R. § 411.354(c)(2).

51. 42 C.F.R. § 411.357(p).

52. 42 C.F.R. § 411.351 (defining "referral").

53. 42 C.F.R. § 411.355(d).

54. 42 C.F.R. § 411.355(g). The list of drugs covered by this exception is updated annually and published on the CMS web site. 42 C.F.R. § 411.355(g). The arrangement for administration or dispensation of the drug must not violate the Anti-Kickback Law. 42 C.F.R. § 411.355(g)(2). Moreover, billing and claim submission for the drugs must be completed in accord with federal and state law. 42 C.F.R. § 411.355(g)(3).

55. 42 C.F.R. § 411.355(h). The list of preventive tests, immunizations, and vaccines covered by this exception is updated annually and published on the CMS web site. 42 C.F.R. § 411.355(h)(5). The arrangement for provision of these items must not violate the Anti-Kickback Law. 42 C.F.R. § 411.355(h)(3). Moreover, billing and claim submission must be completed in accord with federal and state law. 42 C.F.R. § 411.355(h)(4).

56. 42 C.F.R. § 411.355(i). The arrangement for the furnishing of the eyeglasses and contact lenses must not violate the Anti-Kickback Law. 42 C.F.R. § 411.355(i)(2). Moreover, billing and claim submission must be completed in accord with federal and state law. 42 C.F.R. § 411.355(i)(3).

57. 42 C.F.R. § 411.355(f). The arrangement for provision of the implants must not violate the Anti-Kickback Law. 42 C.F.R. § 411.355(f)(3). Moreover, billing and claim submission must be completed in accord with federal and state law. 42 C.F.R. § 411.355(f)(4).

58. 42 U.S.C. § 1395nn(b)(3); 42 C.F.R. § 411.355(c).

59. 42 U.S.C. § 1395nn(d)(2). For purposes of this exception, the term "rural" means an area designated as rural for purposes of calculating the standardized amount for hospitals located in the area under the Medicare inpatient prospective payment system for acute care hospitals. 42 U.S.C. § 1395nn(d)(2).

60. 42 U.S.C. § 1320a-7(b)(8).

61. 42 U.S.C. § 1320a-7a(a)(6). See also OIG Advisory Opinion 01-16 at 4.

62. For purposes of this section, we assume that tax-exempt bonds issued by an exempt hospital qualify for exemption on the basis that they are 501(c)(3) bonds.

63. IRC § 103(a); Treas. Reg. § 1.145-1(a).

64. FY99 CPE at 155.

65. IRC §§ 103(b), 141(e)(1)(G); Treas. Reg. § 1.145-1(a).

66. IRC § 145(a)(1); Treas. Reg. § 1.145-2(b)(3). Portions of a facility owned and used by an exempt hospital in furtherance of its charitable purpose may also be used by nonexempt persons, but only that portion of a "mixed-use facility" owned and used by the hospital may be financed with exempt funds. PLR 9125050 (March 29, 1991); PLR 8827065 (April 14, 1988). The Service has recognized a number of accounting methods to apportion the exempt and nonexempt use of the facility to identify the portion that may be financed with tax-exempt bonds (e.g., allocation by square foot, fair market value, or per procedure). See PLR 9125050 (March 29, 1991); PLR 8827065 (April 14, 1988).

67. IRC § 145(a)(2); Treas. Reg. § 1.145-2(b)(1)-(2). For purposes of this requirement, "net proceeds" are aggregate proceeds from the bond issuance (including proceeds used to pay for the cost of the bond issuance) less amounts maintained in a limited reserve fund. IRC § 148(d). The average maturity on an issue of 501(c)(3) bonds generally may not exceed 120% of the expected economic life of the facilities financed with proceeds from the issue. IRC § 147(b). Finally, there are restrictions on tax arbitrage of bond proceeds as well as procedural requirements for registering and securing public approval for the issuance of such bonds. See IRC §§ 147(f), 148, 149(a), 149(e).

68. IRC § 145(a)(2); Treas. Reg. § 1.145-2(b)(1)-(2).

69. Treas. Reg. § 1.141-3(a).

70. IRC § 103(b). Such interest will also likely be factored into computation of the bondholder's alternative minimum tax. IRC § 57.

71. IRC § 150(b)(3)(A).

72. IRC § 150(b)(3)(B).

73. FY99 CPE at 157.

74. Treas. Reg. §§ 1.141-12, 1.150-4; Rev. Proc. 93-17 (Feb. 19, 1993)

75. Treas. Reg. § 1.145-2(b) (cross referencing Treas. Reg. § 1.141-3(a)-(b)); IR 90-60 (Jan. 2, 1990).

76. Treas. Reg. § 1.145-2(b) (cross referencing Treas. Reg. § 1.141-3(a)-(b)); Rev. Proc. 97-13 (Jan. 10, 1997).

77. IRC § 4958(f)(3); Treas. Reg. § 53.4958-3(b)(2)(i)(B).

78. See supra Chapter 3 of this guide.

79. IRC § 4958(f)(3); Treas. Reg. § 53.4958-3(b)(2)(i)(B).

80. DOJ/FTC Health Industry Guidelines §§ 4-6.

81. DOJ/FTC Health Industry Guidelines §§ 5(B), 6(B).

82. DOJ/FTC Health Industry Guidelines §§ 5, 6.

83. DOJ/FTC Collaboration Guidelines § 3.34.

84. DOJ/FTC Collaboration Guidelines § 3.34.

85. DOJ/FTC Health Industry Guidelines § 9.

86. DOJ/FTC Health Industry Guidelines § 9.

87. DOJ/FTC Health Industry Guidelines § 9(A).

88. DOJ/FTC Health Industry Guidelines § 9(A).

89. DOJ/FTC Health Industry Guidelines § 9(A).

90. DOJ/FTC Health Industry Guidelines § 9(A).

91. FTC Advisory Opinion regarding MedSouth, Inc.(Feb. 19, 2002).

92. DOJ/FTC Health Industry Guidelines § 9(B)(2)(a).

93. DOJ/FTC Health Industry Guidelines § 9(B)(2)(a). DOJ/FTC will look behind the terms of the network agreement in making this inquiry. Thus, if network providers are exclusively (or almost exclusively) furnishing their services through the network, the network will be deemed exclusive even if exclusivity is disclaimed in the network affiliation agreement. DOJ Health Industry Guidelines § 9(B)(2)(a). Moreover, DOJ/FTC will apply the same scrutiny when reviewing restrictions on the ability of a network provider to furnish services outside of the network, even when such restrictions fall short of outright exclusivity. DOJ/FTC Health Industry Guidelines § 9(B)(2)(a).

94. DOJ/FTC Health Industry Guidelines § 9(B)(2)(a)-(b).

95. DOJ/FTC Health Industry Guidelines § 9(C).

96. DOJ/FTC Health Industry Guidelines § 9(C).

97. DOJ/FTC Health Industry Guidelines § 9(C).

98. DOJ/FTC Health Industry Guidelines § 9(C).

Index